MOVE WILD

MOVE WILD

By

ALEXANDRA MERISOIU

ISBNs
978-1-80227-094-5 (paperback)
978-1-80227-095-2 (eBook)

CONTENTS

DISCLAIMER

Same results are not guaranteed and it depends on your condition and whether you have your therapist's permission to exercise. The author is not a licensed medical care provider and has no expertise in diagnosing, examining, or treating medical conditions or injuries of any kind, or in determining the effect of any specific exercise on a medical condition or injury. You should understand that when participating in any exercise or exercise programme, there is the possibility of physical injury. If you engage in the exercise or exercise programmes presented in this book and online resources, you agree that you do so at your own risk, are voluntarily participating in these activities and/or exercises, assume all risk of injury to yourself, and agree to release and discharge the author from any and all claims or causes of action, known or unknown, arising out of following the information in this book and related resources.

ACKNOWLEDGEMENTS

No one ever succeeds alone and I have been lucky to be surrounded by many people who supported me in my lifelong development and helped me to get where I am today, leading to the creation of this book.

I find this section the most difficult to write because the list of people to thank is long, and I wish to leave no one out! The reason for this being difficult is that in this book I seek to distil the ideas that come from the lifelong lessons gathered from all my coaches and instructors, as well as knowledge gained over countless hours of study and research on topics ranging from running biomechanics to myofascial therapy, functional exercise and Alexander Technique; from courses on topics such as Personal Training (PT), physical activity and lifestyle strategies for managing low back pain, training systems courses, and Applied Movement Neurology (AMN); and most importantly from years of personal practice and experimentation and the application of that knowledge in learning to truly understand the mechanics of the human body at a much deeper level.

I would like to thank all my clients, for choosing me as their personal trainer. Our bodies are our most precious assets, and thus I am grateful for the opportunity to lead the way in their personal training and for being entrusted with something so precious and important to each individual. As much as I have taught them, I also have gained valuable lessons from them and have been able to apply all that knowledge and ideas to practice. I would like to thank everyone who shaped, inspired and supported me, each in their own way and thus were part of this journey of mine. I would like to thank my closest family and dear friends who have always been there for me.

I would like to thank my parents for taking me to my first karate lesson. That is when my journey started towards a lifelong passion, hard work and dedication in physical training, leading me to become a Shotokan Karate champion, competing and winning what now seem like countless competitions.

I stepped into a Martial Arts Dojo for the first time at the age of 8 back in 1995 in Romania, at AIKO Club Bucharest. My then Sensei, Aurel Patru, Shihan at the time of writing, was the first coach to introduce me to health, fitness and meditation and he kept pushing me to challenge my limits over the decade I trained with him. I am very grateful for the discipline he instilled in me and the knowledge he shared with me from the early days.

Since then, I also engaged in a variety of other sports and disciplines such as Daito-Ryu Aiki-Jujutsu, Ninjutsu, swimming, rock climbing, yoga, Chi Kung and even Latin American dancing among many others. All sports and disciplines were taught by excellent instructors who also contributed a lot to my knowledge and who shaped me on my personal development journey. Each discipline contributed to the understanding of the human body and the mind. Every movement concerns biomechanics, and interacting with so many people teaches and gives a lot of valuable insight on the topic.

Once I moved to the UK, I qualified as a Personal Trainer and started training with Michael Cohen as his student and client. Michael Cohen was then the founder of Wild Forest Gym. I am grateful for his teachings and for sparking my interest in biomechanics, natural movement and minimalist running. During the time with him, I began to understand a lot about the body and I also trained for Obstacle Course Racing, which was an amazing experience and is a sport I look forward to returning to as a competitor.

Upon joining Shotokan Karate Centres England (SKCE), I met many other instructors who are highly educated and together have enriched my knowledge. I want to thank Sensei Robin from SKCE for supporting and training me for many years. He instilled in me a high level of confidence and self-esteem, which materialised through all the competitions I won when I started to compete for England. It was these wins that brought me the majority of the medals and trophies I won from competing at national and international levels. Since the beginning of my competitive career in Martial Arts, I won close to 100 podium places. Had it not been for Covid and all the cancelled competitions, I am confident that number could have been 100 or more by now.

Most wholeheartedly I would like to thank my mother for her lifetime dedication and support. She devotedly stood by me every step of the way in my journey to becoming who I am today. For giving her all to make sure I had the best education as well as for supporting me in my business endeavour from its conception, for having faith in me and encouraging me to take on any challenges I set for myself with courage and confidence, especially as it was a scary and difficult decision to leave a secure job to start my own business.

I would also like to thank my beloved cousin Alexandra and my aunt Maria for standing by me from the conception of my business, for doing all they could to support me and for investing and believing in me and my success.

Thank you to Richard Matheson for sticking by me since the beginning of my Personal Training career and for helping me grow the business. Richard always encourages me to write and share my knowledge, and this book would likely not have come about had it not been for him continuously encouraging me to share my knowledge with the world.

I would also like to thank Amanda C. Watts and Matthew Watts, from Oompf Global. Amanda was my first business coach. She helped me get the business off the ground and to build it until I could eventually fly on my own. I will be forever grateful for your coaching, support and friendship.

Thanks also to Amelia Balyn, without whom it would have been very difficult to finish this book, for standing by me even when I was stressed and upset at times, and also for helping me with the photography in this book. The photoshoot took 3 back to back weekends to complete and a number of weekends to edit. It was not an easy feat.

There are many complex and dynamic elements to a person's success and a lot of it comes down to other people whom I thank here for being on this beautiful journey with me leading to this book, which I am very excited to share with you.

INTRODUCTION

It goes without saying that behind every success story lie numerous failures to which I was not immune, and there were many! The key to my philosophy is to keep going, whatever I set myself to achieve, taking it one day at a time, but taking it!

Even if it is minimal, I find there is always something I can do towards my goal, and I strongly believe it all adds up and it all counts, especially when it comes to physical training and maintaining the health of your body. I believe in the endless struggle, and although this is what I seek to convey in my work, Move Wild is much more than that. Move Wild is not a competitive sport, it is a lifestyle. Your only competition is you against yourself, one day at a time and your trophy is a healthy body and an enriched and joyful soul. This comes from mindful and meaningful movement, by getting back to and moving in unison with nature.

I began being very passionate about natural movement fitness because it helped me with structural damage in my knees, a result of many years of incorrect training. Structural damage cannot be fully undone, and although I was told I would never heal, since I started practising the exercises I am sharing with you in this book, the pain I used to experience has gone away entirely. The very rare moments when I am aware of it are when my body is telling me off as a result of exercise movements done carelessly, incorrectly or in a way that is damaging in the long run.

This is the reason I want to share this method of exercise with you, because I strongly believe it can help you not only get fit and strong but also reduce the risk of injuries and assist in speeding up recovery time. Gym fitness these days focuses on isolated muscle exercises, forgetting that there is much more to our bodies, and it all matters. The underlying principle of natural movement is the focus on slow twitch muscles across the entire body, in hard-to-reach locations. We don't tend to think about these muscles but they form the basic structural building blocks of our bodies and which we rely on most in our day-to-day lives.

Think of it like yoga mixed with callisthenics, using your natural bodyweight and elements found in nature as props, such as logs and rocks.

Move Wild is for people who believe that there is more to looking after their bodies than just calorie counting. It truly goes to the heart of your inner health and strength from within. Here, I share the knowledge I have gained not only since becoming a Personal Trainer (PT) but from the very first day of I stepped into a Karate Dojo, in 1995. I could not put everything into one book, and there is more to come in the next Move Wild books which I cannot wait to share with you.

I have put my heart into this book, which reflects, I believe, a new philosophy about movement and exercise and a different way of living to what we are used to. This is a technical book in which I not only show you how to do the exercises step by step, but also reveal the underlying reasons for them and explain why they are good for you. This is a manual for your physical development rather than a book you read and put away.

Move Wild builds strength, stamina, mobility and flexibility, it improves posture and balance and brings out the best in you. It strives to educate you on the fundamentals of human movement and body mechanics. It brings precision and sharpness into your training routine, making it more effective and enabling you to reach your goals with less risk of injury and more strength, power and confidence. Move Wild can provide standalone physical training sessions or supplement and alternate with your current routines.

As a business, Move Wild Academy is the evolution of The Merisoiu Technique Institute (MTI) of Health & Human Movement and Urban Women Fitness. It all started with Urban Women Fitness back in 2014, which then evolved into MTI. MTI now focuses primarily on running technique and Move Wild Academy, born back in 2018, brings in the element of primal movements.

Although there are a handful of brand names, the philosophy is the same and the mission is clearer than ever:

To challenge the current fitness paradigm of reps and sets, speed and sweat, through meaningful and mindful primal movement.

After beginning my journey as a Personal Trainer (PT) it didn't take long for me to realise that classic gym PT, based on exercises that don't incorporate a lot of movement and are repeated in sets and reps, was not the way to go for me. Coming from a solid Martial Arts background with almost three decades of training experience and intense competition, I was developing a different coaching style and training approach. From the start, the idea of classic exercises reps and sets did not sit well with my preference for meaningful practice, as in Martial Arts or Yoga.

Move Wild is not simply about fitness and exercise, it is about continuous and gradual improvement at a deeper level and in a more meaningful way: the Move Wild way. The exercises can still be performed in sets and reps, but there is more substance, more movement and more purpose behind them.

The term 'meaningful' is subjective, so what does it mean to you? Perhaps you are looking to have more freedom of movement? Moving with less pain, with more comfort and confidence? Or perhaps you are looking for robust all-round fitness and the ability to truly perform whatever physical challenges you set yourself? Perhaps your aim is to be more mindful, connect with your body and the world around you? Or perhaps you simply want to spend more time in nature, be it alone or with others around you.

Whatever a meaningful exercise means to you, perhaps Move Wild could become something meaningful for you?

True inner health and strength is developed over time, one day at a time. How much effort and time you dedicate to a continuous routine, I leave for you to decide. Our lifestyles and needs differ and we are the best judges of what feels right and works best for us. As a guideline I would advise to have a training routine in place at least 3 days of the week, either exclusively Move Wild or with Move Wild as supplementing other routines.

I went beyond the classic Personal Training systems, because my clients wanted to get strong and fit. For that, they first need to understand how their bodies function in order to move fluidly but with strength and confidence, much like a panther. More importantly, they need to learn to prevent and manage injuries, and become mindful of their movements and of moving with purpose.

It is essential not to sacrifice mindful movement for sets, reps and speed. It is imperative to understand the difference between tension and relaxation, intentional movement, posture, balance and counterbalance, as these are the foundations upon which a strong structure can be built. The more aware one becomes of how the body moves in space and how it feels, the more control and confidence in movement one develops.

It became clear to me that my clients needed a complete, all-round system which would offer them the foundations they needed to live a healthy, strong and fit life. By understanding the basics of human movement, posture, breathing, nutrition and mindful control, we can take control of our own health and fitness. This is the philosophy behind my work which I will attempt to pass down to you in this book. I will not touch on nutrition here, but you might see a future book on this topic.

Much too often the focus is placed on how many times an exercise is repeated, rather than aiming at correct form with fewer repetitions. Doing an exercise mindfully to your best ability is much more effective and efficient, as you get the correct muscles working. It is easy to drift away in thoughts while exercising, perhaps planning a dinner, and some of us will even have something to watch while working out. To truly give your body and mind the exercise they need, remaining mindful is key as it truly engages the nervous system.

That being said, reps, sets and speed do have their time and place. They come after mastering the correct form and technique and once the concepts of body alignment, bodyweight distribution and stability muscles are understood. In this book you will learn about these fundamental principles of human movement and you will begin to understand the benefits Move Wild exercises could have for you and your body.

Move Wild Academy methods stem from a combination of disciplines: Martial Arts, primarily Shotokan Karate, as well as Daito-Ryu, dancing, climbing, the POSE Method of running, Ido Portal and MovNat. Move Wild encompasses knowledge from multiple sources and it does not restrict itself to a narrow vision. Inspired by all these different methods of training, I immersed myself in studying human body mechanics and in trying and testing various methods of movement to get to the bottom of their potential benefits. All this, combined with discussions with physiotherapists and chiropractors, led me to a deeper understanding of the human body, which now enables me to share and pass this knowledge on to you.

So what does meaningful movement mean to you? What does moving with purpose tell you? By reading this book you will already have expanded your awareness, and if you practice some of the exercises, you will have taken a great step towards your goals.

The exercises in this book come with accompanying videos. To access them, head to www.movewildacademy.com/move-wild and enter the password "duck-walk".

Enjoy the exercises and share your stories and wild moments with me on social media using #MoveWild.

Alexandra

CHAPTER 1. MOVE WILD PHILOSOPHY

Move Wild is as much an educational system as it is a physical training system. This book has been created for both purposes.

At its core, Move Wild values technique over speed. Once technique is learnt you move on to performing the movement for a longer time, keeping the form as correct as possible. You fully immerse yourself into the movement and the practice. When you can hold the form for long enough then you can introduce speed and perform the movement at a faster pace. This is where you receive the cardiovascular benefits of Move Wild. However, always return to slow, mindful and technical movements even when you get to the advanced phase. When speeding up, technique breaks down and imbalances begin to creep in, and if left unchallenged over long periods of time, they add up and could potentially lead to overuse injuries.

Gradual progress is key to developing the body and reducing the risk of injuries. It also makes the practice enjoyable and not a burden as you progress through each stage and begin to observe the benefits. Depending on your fitness level, you will progress slower or faster. The speed at which you make progress is not important, what is important is to allow your body to adapt to a different type of movement you might never have attempted before. Remember, Move Wild improves your mobility and flexibility while building strength. If you are not very flexible or very strong, you need to give your muscles, ligaments, tendons, fascia and skeletal system time to adapt and absorb the new movements and changes.

It's interesting how we have one body for a lifetime, which we cannot change, but we take greater care of our cars which we can change anytime. To a certain extent you are your best coach and doctor. When practised as it should be, Move Wild will teach you how to connect with your own body and breath. You will be challenged to mentally scan your body and identify what muscles are being used andto feel your body inside and out. To feel connected with your body and your breath.

If you have ever practised Martial Arts, ballet, golf or almost any other sport that has an artful component, then you will recognise that Move Wild is taught and practised as you would practise an art. Anyone can exercise, but not everyone has the base level of movement capacity to perform movement patterns in a healthy and efficient way. This is true for running as well. Everyone can run, but how they run dictates how much they expose themselves to injuries and the level of performance they can reach. Practise with detail in mind, with passion in your movement and always be aware of what you are doing and how and what you are feeling.

Move Wild exercises are low impact and put little to no strain on joints, some movements less or more than others. Thus it is possible for almost anyone to safely perform the movements to get stronger and improve flexibility and mobility.

The aim of Move Wild is to educate and empower readers to be able to coach themselves if they wish to. Our mission is to inform and encourage independent study of physical movement and expression.

Finally, Move Wild, at its core, encompasses Zanshin. Zanshin is the Japanese term for awareness or relaxed awareness. This brings the meaningful and mindful component into your Move Wild practice.

THE MOVE WILD PYRAMID

The Move Wild pyramid depicts the phases one follows when learning to move mindfully and meaningfully. There is no defined and precise boundary between stages. They all interconnect with each other. But for the purpose of understanding the Move Wild training philosophy we will present each stage as a separate part.

FLOW PHASE
Mastery level.
Perform sequences of
exercises with good technique
and fluid transitions, for a longer
time. Flow from one to another.

SPEED PHASE
Advanced level. Perform the exercise for a long
time and at speed while maintaining form.

ENDURANCE PHASE
Intermediate level. Perform the exercise for
longer periods of time, over a longer distance.
Perform repetitions while maintaining form.

DEEP PRACTICE
Fundamentals or beginner's level. Focus on form and deep
practice. this is your mindful practice phase.

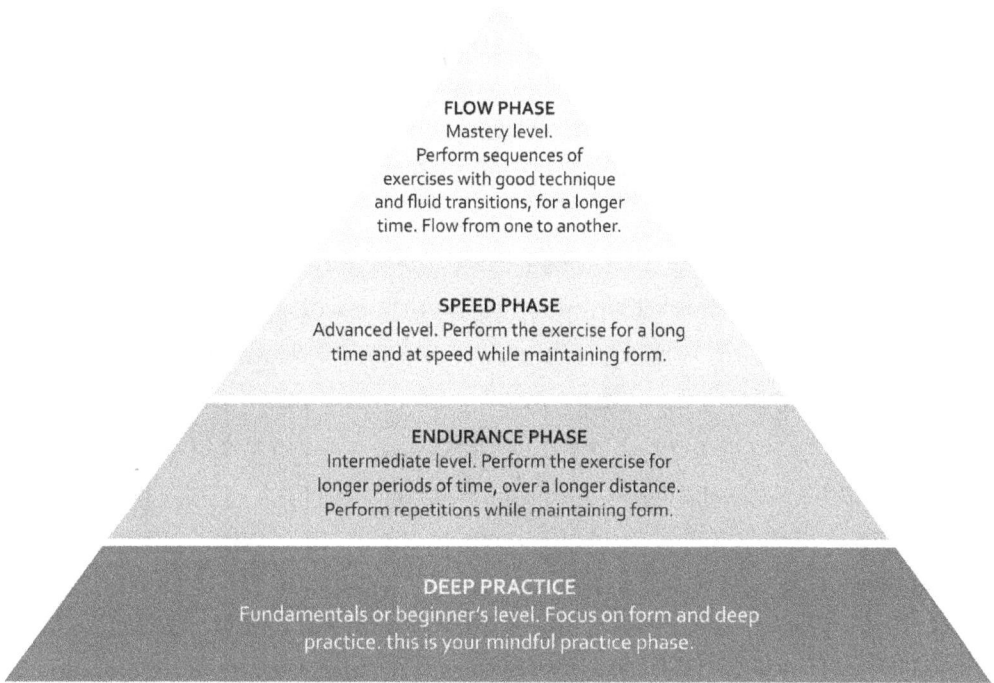

Move Wild Pyramid

1. Deep practice

This is the first and most important phase of the Move Wild training system. Deep practice is about building the foundations for efficient movement. This is where you learn and become aware of your body, how it functions, what it needs and how to work with the muscles. This is also the stage where elite athletes learn the movements.

I encourage you take your time, move slowly, and feel the movement in your body. There is no rush to get anywhere. This is the "technical" stage when you focus your attention on the details of the movement, receive feedback and correct what needs to be corrected. It's not about sets and reps or going fast and sweating a lot. This stage is about exploring movement and learning the techniques. This is also in line with Deliberate Practice, a term used by Anders Ericsson in his book

Peak[1]. This is how elite athletes become great at what they do. Move Wild adopts a similar process.

At the end of the exercise I encourage you to take 10 seconds as your break, and ask yourself the question: *Where in my body do I feel the exercise?*

This will give you an idea of whether you performed the exercise correctly and where you rweaknesses lie, which you could then address. It can also be beneficial for you to understand which muscles should be working when performing a certain movement. This is how you learn to focus and activate the correct muscles at will. Most of Move Wild is about you learning this, about your own body and experience. Make it meaningful movement by being mindful and knowing why and how you perform a movement in the first place. This way your practice is effective, yielding the results you want.

I encourage you to move slowly and with absolute control. This is when you truly engage your muscles and become stronger to the deepest layers. Think about the exercises physiotherapists prescribe to patients. Those exercises are slow to begin with, and with control. This is true strength. There should be minimal aggressive push off against the ground, thumping on landing or side swaying of the hips (depending on the exercise). Think about setting sail in a boat. You can sit in the boat and push off against the dock behind you or you can tie a rope to the front of the boat and pull it away from the dock. With Move Wild exercises, you want to use your core to pull your feet off the ground rather than pushing off against the ground. There is some push off which cannot be avoided, but it should be reduced as much as possible. By engaging with the content of the book and the online resources, you will develop control over your body and movement. This control comes from your core and hips, and mastering your body in this way will help you to reduce injuries, build strength and gain movement confidence.

If you are not convinced, Newton's third law states that for every action there is an equal and opposite reaction. Thus the harder you push against the ground, the more the ground will respond with a similar level of aggressiveness. If you are gentler, you will receive a more gentle response.

---

1 Ericsson, A. and Pool, R., 2017. *Peak*. Vintage.

The push off theory doesn't just apply to Move Wild ground-based exercises but also to running and jumping.

When you engage in Move Wild training I encourage you to breathe on each movement and, with the relevant exercises, to breathe out on the effort. There will be guidance on breathing later in the book.

To measure your progress you can:

- Rate the level of difficulty on a scale of 1 to 10 based on how you feel; this is subjective measuring
- Keep track of how long it takes until you lose your form
- Count how many steps or reps you can perform until you lose your form

While you can measure your progress in various ways, there should be no pressure to perform a certain number of sets and reps at this stage or for a certain period of time.

2. Endurance phase

After you practise the fundamentals and have a good degree of control (this comes sooner or later depending on the individual) you can perform the exercises for longer periods while still maintaining the form as best you can.

How do you know when you are ready? When you begin to feel stronger when you do the Panther Walk or have more balance when you do the Clock. If you start from scratch, 8–10 training session should be enough for you to move to the endurance phase. If you are fitter and used to such movements, 5–7 sessions will do.

Although Move Wild is not about sets and reps, these can be introduced at this stage, as well as distance for progress measurement. However, I recommend you not to emphasise sets and reps as it can lead to you wanting to perform the number at the cost of technique.

3. Speed phase

After you have gained the strength, control and endurance to perform the movements at a good level you can perform the movements faster while trying as much as possible to hold on to your form and your breathing.

At speed, form will eventually break down. The challenge is to keep the form as correct as possible for as long as possible and at a gradually faster pace.

Again this stage can come sooner or later for each individual. In fact I introduce the cardio sessions at the end of workouts very early for most of my clients after they practise the technical aspect at the beginning of the sessions. Even a 10 minutes circuit using the movements you have just learnt in the main session will be enough for Move Wild beginners. If you are more experienced, go for 20–30 minutes at the end of your deep practice. If you are unsure, stick to technique and endurance and then slowly introduce the 5 minutes of cardio at the end.

If you are recovering from injuries or don't have the strength just yet and you rate the exercise difficulty high in deep practice, introduce the speed stage later.

4. Flow phase

This stage is for more experienced Move Wild practitioners. You now have a good understanding of technique, good fitness levels and a library of movements to choose from.

It's time to create a flow of movements by yourself. This is a more advanced level of deep practice.

In the end you develop movements and reflexes and the body is prepared to react with strength, balance and control whenever you need it to (i.e. on the mat while wrestling, on the street or at home if tripping or slipping).

Enjoy this stage as you can flow from one movement to another without planning ahead.

THE MOVE WILD PRACTICE

Now that we've got the theory out of the way, let's move closer to the practical part of Move Wild.

The Move Wild curriculum also includes jumping technique, running technique, falling technique and lifting and throwing technique. However, this book deals with body weight training only, to build strength, flexibility, agility, improve your balance and reduce the risk of injuries.

Move Wild exercises work in all 3 planes of motion – sagittal, frontal and transverse – and train the body as a whole unit. You will learn more about the 3 planes of motion later in the book.

In this book we will be looking at the following:

A. Fundamentals
    1. The core
    2. Breathing
    3. The tripod
    4. The bucket of water
    5. Alignment
    6. Elongating the body
    7. Clenching vs tucking
    8. Synovial fluid

B. Warmup
    1. Cardio
    2. Fluid Stretch
    3. Fascia Stretches

C. More Wild Exercises
    1. Strength
        a. Full Squat
        b. Panther Walk
        c. Crab Walk
        d. Frog Jump Spot
        e. Frog Jump Forwards
        f. Frog Jump Side

g. Frog Jump Twisted

h. Frog Leap

i. Tiger Walk

j. The Crocodile

k. Duck Walk

l. Split Squat

m. Cross Frog

n. Side Monkey

o. Bunny Hop

2. Balance and stability

a. The Clock

b. 360 Degrees

c. Seesaw

d. Standing Body Weight Transfer

e. Prone Body Weight Transfer

f. Supine Body Weight Transfer

g. Prone to Supine Flow

3. Stretches

a. Stretches

b. Lizard

c. Pigeon

d. Side Kick Frog

e. Gorilla

CHAPTER 2. MOVE WILD FUNDAMENTALS

In this chapter we will briefly go through the fundamentals of Move Wild. Each element has its own chapter and I have written numerous articles on them. In this book we focus on the movements themselves and understanding these 8 fundamental principles as they are very important for movement in general.

The 8 fundamentals of Move Wild are:

1. The core
2. Breathing
3. The tripod
4. The bucket of water
5. Alignment
6. Elongating the body
7. Clenching vs tucking
8. Synovial fluid

THE CORE

The core of your body, or the trunk, consists of the abdominal muscles, sides of the abdomen, the back and the pelvis, and it goes all the way up to the diaphragm.

Understanding how to activate, or rather control, your core is one of the most important steps in your development. This is the foundation for your physical strength. That's because all movement comes from your core, so controlling the core means you will have better control over your body.

Once you manage to connect with your core and focus on building strength in that area you will gain:

1. Power

Core strength is the foundation for powerful, explosive movements such as jumping, sprinting and throwing. All movement begins from your core and your core supports the rest of your body and the execution of the movement itself.

2. Back health

Most people will experience low back pain at some stage in their life. "Experts estimate that up to 80% of the population will experience back pain at some time in their lives."[2]

"Most cases of back pain are mechanical or non-organic – meaning they are not caused by serious conditions, such as inflammatory arthritis, infection, fracture or cancer."[3]

Your back pain affects your posture, level of activity, degree of flexibility, stretch, core strength, injuries and so on. It is recommended to "stay active"[4] when experiencing acute non-specific lower back pain.

A strong core is essential to a healthy back that will carry your body throughout your life. So keep your core strong. Move Wild focuses on developing your core strength with each and every exercise. Part of the body will not move in isolation while practising Move Wild because it never moves in isolation in your daily routine either.

---

2 *Back Pain Facts and Statistics*. American Chiropractic Association. Available at: www.acatoday.org/Patients/What-is-Chiropractic/Back-Pain-Facts-and-Statistics

3 *Back Pain Facts and Statistics*. American Chiropractic Association. Available at: www.acatoday.org/Patients/What-is-Chiropractic/Back-Pain-Facts-and-Statistics

4 NHS.uk. 2020. *Back pain*. Available at: www.nhs.uk/conditions/back-pain/

3. Balance

If you ever find yourself in a situation in which your balance or stability are compromised, a strong core will come to the rescue.

A strong core leads to better balance and improved movement confidence. Remember, all movement comes from the core, including your reflexes and balance.

4. Reduce risk of injuries

Walking, running, balance, lifting, carrying, throwing, and catching are all movements we do throughout our lives. A strong core will give you a better chance of fewer injuries and of living without pain. This is because every part of your body has its job to do. Your core supports your body in motion. If your core is weak, its job needs to be taken on by a different part of the body and this leads to compensation.

The part of your body that takes on more work because of your weak core, let's say the quads for example, will eventually fatigue and start to be exposed to injuries.

There is no doubt that having a strong core will enable you to build the lasting foundations required for a fit, healthy, strong and powerful body, but how do we work with it? How do we actively, or intentionally engage our core and not just wait for it to happen?

How to activate or engage your core muscles

There are a few ways to explain what engaging or activating your core means and how to achieve it. I have learnt to explain this one action in various ways because not all my clients understood what engage your core meant, or how to tense your core by using your breathing.

1. Breathing

Learning deep breathing has many other benefits besides activating the core, but for now we focus just on this. Pulling your stomach muscles in as you breathe out is the first step towards learning how to activate your core muscles. As you breathe out, your abdominal muscles pull in (your abdomen deflates like a balloon) and the whole core activates, or tenses.

Later in this book you will learn more about deep breathing, its benefits and breathing exercises.

2. Brace for punching

You are not really getting punched of course. Just pretend someone is trying to punch you in the stomach. What would you do? How would you react if you had to "receive" a punch? You'd brace for the punch, trying to withstand the blow. You'd also notice that when you brace for a punch, you breath out slightly and direct the belly button towards the back of the body.

3. Lying on the ground

Lie on the ground – preferably a hard, flat surface – face up, with your knees bent and feet flat on the ground. Notice the natural curve in your lower back. Now try to flatten your lower back, touching the ground with the portion of your spine in the lower back. You will notice that to do this, you need to tense your abdominal muscles.

4. Sucking the stomach in

Sucking the stomach in is another way to describe the core activation process. However, when you suck your stomach in, you don't necessarily tense your abdominal muscles, maybe just a little, but not enough. This is one way used by trainers to coach their trainees, but not the first method I tend to use. When you exercise, you might find it easier to think about tensing the abdominal muscles when you want to activate your core. It's easier to visualise, feel and control. But remember that your core includes more than just your abdomen.

BREATHING

The way you breathe is an important part of the MoveWild training. Once you have understood the physical movement, pattern or form, the outer layer of the exercise itself, then you can focus on more subtle elements such as breathing patterns.

If you start focusing on how you breathe before you learn the fundamental movements, your technique will suffer. Don't worry, you'll still be learning about breathing but your focus will be primarily on the movement to begin with.

As a general rule, when performing an exercise think about:

* breathing out on the effort
* maintaining a smooth, unrestricted breathing flow (i.e. don't hold your breath)
* breathing deeply

According to Michael Cohen from RaphaYad Bioenergy Treatment School, shallow breathing may lead to:

* Not fully emptying and filling the lungs, thus pushing stale air around the body.
* Cardiovascular limitations. The heart may feel the strain of certain physical actions such as running, strength training, weight lifting, sports and even just a walk down the road.
* Reverse breathing (i.e. stomach moves in when breathing in and out when breathing out), therefore it could be putting strain on the breathing mechanism and restricting the amount of oxygen when under stress, strain or pressure.

Potential benefits that can be achieved by incorporating deep breathing exercises into your day are:

19

- Emptying lungs. This ensures that air circulates throughout the area.
- Improving the circulatory system.
- Increasing the amount of oxygen in the blood.
- Improving the cardiovascular system. The heart is a muscle and can be developed with practice.
- Can direct the breath into areas of the body where there are injuries and illnesses. This stimulates healing as well as calming down stress or anxiety.
- Contributing to your warmup before exercise.
- Reducing the required recovery period after exercise.

Checking for Reverse breathing

Many people reverse breathe without realising and without causing a problem. Others may struggle when under physical strain, physical exercise, stress or anxiety. In order to check, complete the following breathe test:

- Place one hand over the stomach and one over the chest.
- Take a deep long breathe in and out through nose, keeping the mouth closed. Make sure that the in and out breathes are the same length.
- Observe whether the hand on the stomach moves in or out with the in breath and the out breathe. The hand on the chest should not be moving.
- If your stomach moves in when you breath in and out when you breath out, you may be reverse breathing.

Correct breathing

The stomach expands, moving the hand out with the in breath and deflates, moving the hand inwards when you breathe out.

In breath - stomach expands - moving the hand outwards.
Out breathe - stomach deflates - moving the hand inwards.

Reverse breathing is the opposite. When you reverse breathe, it means you are trying to fill up something that is deflating. This is particularly important for those who suffer from pressure, stress and anxiety.

Diaphragmatic breathing

One of the fundamental steps in learning to breathe well is to learn diaphragmatic breathing.

The diaphragm is the dome-shaped sheet of muscle inserted into the lower ribs. It separates the abdominal cavity from the thoracic cavity. The shape of diaphragm is like an upside-down U.

When we inhale, the diaphragm contracts and is drawn down into the abdominal cavity until it is flat.

Simultaneously the external intercostal muscles between the ribs elevate the anterior rib cage.

The stomach expands, because the dome of the diaphragm has flattened, and not because the muscles in the abdominal location have contracted.

During exhalation, the rib cage drops to its resting position while the diaphragm relaxes and elevates to its dome-shaped position in the thorax.

Air within the lungs is forced out of the body as the size of the thoracic cavity decreases.

THE TRIPOD

The foot tripod is like a camera tripod, a stable shape. In the human body this is formed by the big toe, little toe and heel.

If the core is the foundation of your physical strength and everyday movement, the tripod is the foundation of your body, like the foundation of a building upon which all its floors rest.

To help create awareness of the tripod, use the following body weight distribution exercise. You will see this exercise later in the book in more detail.

Step 1: Position your feet hip width apart with toes facing forwards. If the feet are straight, the big toes face inwards slightly.

Step 2: Slowly and smoothly transfer your bodyweight from one foot to the other without lifting either foot off the ground.

Feel the weight moving from one side to the other and the pressure against the ground as each foot in turn takes on more weight.

After a while (take as long as you need to become aware of the bodyweight transfer), stop somewhere in the middle where you feel your weight is evenly distributed on both feet; 50% of your weight on your right foot and 50% on your left foot. Hold this distribution as best you can while moving on to step 3.

Step 3: Slowly and smoothly transfer your bodyweight to the front (ball of the foot) and then to the back (heel) of your feet without lifting the toes or the heels off the ground.

Feel the weight and the pressure against the ground moving from the front to the back of your feet.

After a while (as long as you need to become aware of the bodyweight transfer) stop somewhere in the middle where you feel your weight is evenly distributed on the front and back of your feet; roughly 50% of your weight on the heels and 50% on the balls of the feet.

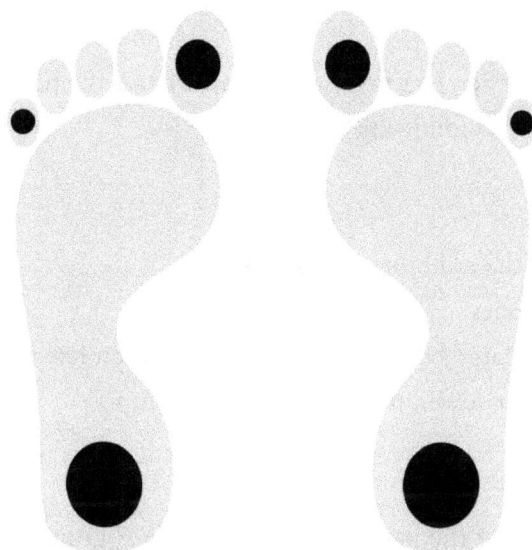

The tripod

You may find it difficult to begin with as you may not have the body awareness needed for such subtleties. However, the more often you attempt to perform this exercise, the better you will become at it. And have patience, with Move Wild patience is essential. Leave all worries and troubles behind and just focus on the moment: there is no wrong or right, there is just attempting and improving.

Once you start developing awareness, you might begin to notice that you are shifting the body weight on the toes too much. Tell yourself to place 51% of your weight on the heels. That should balance your weight more evenly on the tripod. Just 1% is all that's needed to bring awareness to your body.

THE BUCKET OF WATER

Before we go any further, let's first understand what is the hip and what is the pelvis. The pelvis contains the following[5]:

1. Sacrum
2. Coccyx (or the tail bone)
3. Three hip bones
   a. Ilia. The large bones, left and right, you can feel and see.
   b. Pubis. The lower, posterior part of the hip.
   c. Ischium.

So the hips are part of the pelvis. However, while aligning the body, it's alright to think about the large bone you can feel and see, one on each side of the body: the ilium. It's much easier to align thinking about the ilia as they are an easier point of reference than the pelvis.

The pelvis forms a shape like a bucket of water, holding water in it. In fact the pelvis protects your organs and the spinal column. [6]

So why is it important for you to understand how your pelvic bones positioned? Because this is a major element in low back pain, in the strength of your core, in shortening your hip flexors which leads to injuries in the area, as well as in shortened or lengthened hamstrings which make you more prone to injuries. Understanding how to carry your body, which includes understanding the pelvis position, can literally save you a lot of pain.

When you tilt your pelvis forwards, known as an anterior pelvic tilt, you over-arch your lower back and spill water forwards. When this happens your abdominal muscles are not as activated as they should be to support your body and especially your lower back. Thus your lower back and your lumbar spine are tasked with more weight and pressure than they are designed for.

5 Johns Hopkins Medicine. *Pelvis Problems*. Available at: www.hopkinsmedicine.org/health/conditions-and-diseases/pelvis-problems.

6 Johns Hopkins Medicine. *Pelvis Problems*. Available at: www.hopkinsmedicine.org/health/conditions-and-diseases/pelvis-problems.

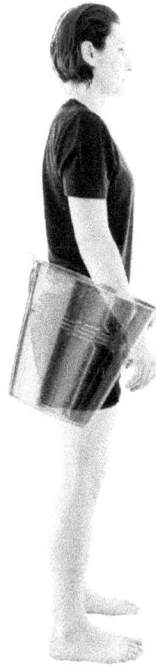

Anterior pelvic tilt

In this position, your hamstrings are weak and underactive, and so are your abdominal muscles and glutes. Moreover, your quadriceps and hip flexors are short, tight and overactive. These underactive and overactive areas can also cause the forward pelvis tilt, so as you can see, it's a vicious cycle.

When you tilt your pelvis backwards, a posterior pelvic tilt, you tuck your tail bone inward/forwards, your belly button looks up towards the sky and your back curves outwards (towards the back). You spill water behind you and the lumbar spine in curved outwards and pressure is being put on the intervertebral discs.

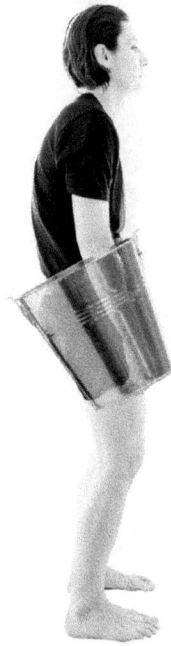

Posterior pelvic tilt

This being said, emphasising the tilting of the pelvis backwards and forwards is actually a good body awareness exercise on its own and it's also good to mobilise the spine and pelvis. This works as long as you are aware of what you are doing and you don't carry your pelvic tilts on a daily basis. So let's practise this easy exercise.

Pelvic tilt exercise

When you tilt your pelvis forwards and backwards, ensure that your upper and lower body stay still as much as possible. There will be some movement in the rest of the body, but it will be minimal. You don't want to slouch as you tilt backwards or push your chest out excessively when tilting forwards.

Also pay attention to your knees, which tend to bend as you tilt the pelvis. This is a common error that comes with this exercise. Keep your knees soft but avoid bending and straightening them excessively.

After performing a few repetitions of the exercise, stop somewhere in the middle of the movement where you feel you aren't spilling water forwards or backwards. This is where you should be all the time, even when sitting. This is the point where your spine is in neutral position and your core and glutes are slightly activated.

This is the whole exercise. There are other versions of it, making it more efficient. But if you do this from time to time alongside the Move Wild exercises, it's really beneficial.

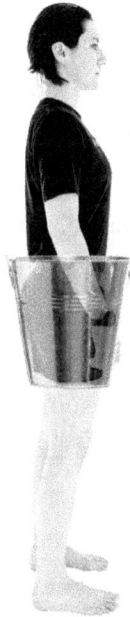

Neutral position

ALIGNMENT

After understanding and practising the fundamental elements – tripod, bucket, core – you can move on to a basic understanding of body alignment. This is, of course, related to the previous ones: the tripod, hip alignment and understanding of the core make up the correct alignment.

Many of the aches and pains we experience may very well come from improper body alignment.

If you understand what may be causing your pain, you will begin to change the way you carry yourself, walk, run, sit and stand and, in time, you will experience less pain and more freedom of movement, which is the essence of Move Wild practice.

This is not a biomechanics book, but rather the purpose of it is to introduce you to the basics of body alignment. Body alignment begins with awareness of your body, how it is positioned and how it should be positioned to enable it to function optimally.

Correct body alignment might feel unnatural to many of us because our bodies have been affected by the modern world and the muscles have adjusted to fit some unnatural positions. Take the foot for example. We are born with toes spread and wide. Modern shoes squish the toes together and we are told that is normal. In reality most modern shoes have damaged our feet. Just because you've got used to it, doesn't mean it's good for you. The "texting neck" is another example, where your head it tilted forwards. You've got used to it and now having proper alignment might feel strange, but that doesn't mean that this head tilt is good for you, in fact it's very detrimental as we will soon see. So let's understand what correct alignment and posture actually look and feel like. We will begin with the feet and make our way up to the head.

1. **Feet alignment**. Place your feet roughly hip width apart, with the outside of the foot pointing forwards and toes facing slightly inwards, this will encourage hip and knee stability and help the muscles to mould around this new position.

    If you look closely, you will notice that your feet are in alignment with the sides of your hips and with your knees. If you have a knee valgus (when your knees collapse in) then the knees and feet won't be in alignment and in this case it's even more important to align your feet properly to avoid unnecessary pressure on the knees. Knee valgus is another story so we will not go into detail here. What we want is to build awareness around body alignment so you know how it should feel.

This doesn't mean you have to walk like this and think about it all the time. No, this awareness is a form of training until it becomes a habit. There should be moments in your day or during your practice when you focus on this particular aspect.

Do this mindful practice on a consistent basis and your body will begin to develop in the way you train it, with improved alignment, reducing stress and tension and allowing your body to move with more freedom. It will also strengthen areas of the body which are weaker due to incorrect alignment and reduce pressure on the areas of the body that work extra for the areas that don't do their job.

So what does this mean to you? It means, with time, patience and practice, your body will be less achy and painful and you will reduce the risk of injuries and early wear and tear.

2. **The tripod**. Each of your feet form a tripod with the big toe, little toe and heel; focus on keeping this tripod on the ground at all times. Go back to the *Tripod* section to review the step by step guide.

3. **Evenly distributed weight.** Use the bodyweight distribution exercise in the *Tripod* section. If you have access to a scale that shows body weight distribution, use it. Keep in mind that your mission is to encourage body awareness, but using technology can make this easier, faster and more interesting. It can help you to understand how even weight distribution actually feels.

    I used one of those scales once and I had to put a bit more weight on my left leg. It felt very unnatural. However, what was unnatural and detrimental was how I was walking regularly, with most of my weight on my right leg. Funnily enough the right side of my body has always been injured and had issues most often. This would explain why, or would at least be an important piece of the puzzle.

    Even weight distribution means distribution between your left and right foot, as well as between the heels and the balls of your feet, as described in the *Tripod* section.

4. **Soft knees**. Prevent your knees from locking (i.e.being fully straightened). However, soft knees doesn't mean bending them either. It's subtle. Try locking your knees and then relaxing them. That's "soft".

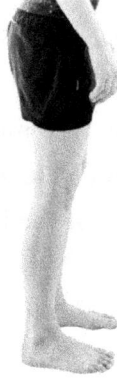

Soft knees

5. **Bucket of water**. Imagine your pelvis as a bucket of water; align your pelvis and feel free to think about the 2 bony protuberant structures as your hips, as this makes it easier to see the alignment. Ensure you don't spill water forwards or backwards. Refer back to the *Bucket of Water* section.

6. **Core**. If your hips (a.k.a. the bucket of water), are aligned, then your core will be slightly contracted or activated. You won't feel a burn but a light tension. Refer back to the *Core* section.

7. **Shoulders.** Align your shoulders with your ears without lifting your chin or tilting your head. Try making a double chin by pushing your head back while keeping your chin parallel to the ground. This is an Alexander Technique method of achieving alignment.

8. **Chin.** The chin should be parallel to the ground and slightly tucked in as if to create a double chin. This places the head and the cervical spine in alignment, in their most natural position with less strain and pressure on the vertebrae. According to Dr Scott Collins, ORA Orthopedics Spine Surgeon, when the

head is tilted forwards, the pressure on your cervical spine increases. You head weighs about 10–12lb (4.5–5.4kg). When you tilt your head forwards at a 15 degree angle, you place about 27lb (12kg) of pressure on your neck. A 30 degree tilt is 40lb (18kg) of pressure and a 45 degree tilt, 49lb (22kg) of pressure[7]. That's a lot of pressure on the vertebrae.

There are a few more detrimental consequences of having the head out of alignment. A forwards tilt of the head places unnecessary strain on the neck muscles, particularly a muscle called the sternocleidomastoid. Moving down towards the shoulders, it can also stretch and strain the trapezius muscles on either side of the neck and finally it stretches and strains the muscles alongside the spine.

What I am also particular about are the nerves that travel from the brain through the cervical spine and down to the rest of the body. The only way for the brain to communicate with the body is through the nervous system. The nervous system must pass through the cervical spine. The nerves protected by the cervical vertebrae then branch off to the organs and extremities, but they must pass through the cervical spine, there is no other way.

Imagine the spine and spinal cord like a hose. Electrical impulses, which contain information passed from the brain to the body, pass through that hose. This could be healing information or a request for energy. If your neck is bent and strained all the time, this communication is impaired and ineffective.

There is also the risk of trapped nerves in the neck and around the trapezius muscles.

This doesn't mean you have to walk around like a robot. This information is meant to bring some awareness to how you carry yourself and perhaps explain why you have aches and pains around the neck in particular, or why you might have had a trapped nerve in the past.

Try to gently stretch your neck regularly to release some of the tension from those over-stretched and strained muscles. Don't mind how strange

---

7 Collins, D. *Heads up! How to Prevent Pain in Your "Text Neck"* ORA Orthopedics. Available at: <www.qcora.com/heads-prevent-pain-text-neck/>.

it looks, tilt your neck left and right anytime and anywhere you need to. I do get some looks when I do it, but then people get used to it. So do what you need to do!

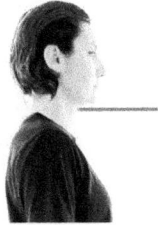

Chin parallel to the ground

9. Imagine a **straight line** from your **ears** to your **shoulders** to your **hips** to the back of your **knee** and just in front of the **ankles** as shown in *Alignment* photo.

10. Imagine a **straight line** from the **nose** to the **solar plexus** to the **belly button.** These three points should be "stacked" on top of each other in your mind and physically.

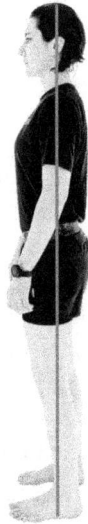

Alignment

When you perform the elongating the body visualisation which follows, you should begin by aligning the body as shown in the Alignment image.

You can also alternate between the body alignment visualisation and the elongating the body visualisation. This depends on the type of workout you are designing (i.e. a balance and body weight transfer session should have both visualisations as part of the session).

ELONGATING THE BODY

Probably the best and most important lesson I was taught when I started learning natural movement was how to align and elongate my body. Elongating the body helps to relax the muscles and release some of the pressure placed on joints.

After you have gone through the alignment   you can use the elongating the body visualisation to fine-tune your body awareness. Repeating these 2 exercises on a regular basis will enable you to develop physical awareness, which, in turn, will help you to perform a wider variety of movements in a more efficient way.

Greater body awareness and control also reduces the risk of injuries. For example, falls lead to injuries, but they don't have to. The greater your body awareness, balance, coordination, strength and mobility, the greater control you have over your falls and this reduces the risk of getting injured. If you also develop your body to be strong in various positions and stances, the risk of injuries again reduces and if they do happen, they won't last as long or be as serious.

The elongating the body visualisation begins at the feet and continues up through the body to the head. You can also begin with the head if you wish. It's good to do this visualisation with your eyes closed, so maybe ask someone to read the following out loud to you or record yourself and listen to it. The instructions are the same as in a meditation, so there is a lot of repetition. Let's begin:

1. Stand with the feet roughly hip width apart, with your toes facing forwards.
2. Ensure your body weight is distributed evenly on the left and right foot and between the balls of your feet and your heels (remember the tripod). The bucket of water is evenly balanced, without spilling any water. The knees are

33

soft throughout. When you elongate your body you only have to imagine and not actually move your body. In fact your body will take the shape of the image you hold in your mind. Don't try too hard, even if you feel you can't get something right, leave it and move on to the next stage.

3. Take a deep breath in through your nose, deep into your abdomen, and exhale through your mouth as you relax your shoulders, arms, elbows, wrists, hands and fingers. Relax your shoulders and allow your shoulder blades to release any tension and widen. Adjust your chin to be parallel to the ground.

4. Now imagine a piece of string attached to the crown of your head and to the ceiling, the sky, a branch or anything above your head. Then take the piece of string down through your body, through your legs, all the way down to your feet. Follow the string with your mind's eye as it lengthens through the body. As you go through the visualisation, use only your imagination. Avoid any actual movement. There is no need for you to take any action. All you need to do is imagine.

5. From the top of your head, take the piece of string and imagine how your ankles elongate away from your feet. Imagine a small space forming between your ankles and your feet. Imagine your bones, muscles, tendons and ligaments having space to breathe and relax. You will do the same for all the joints as you go through.

6. Going up the body, take the piece of string and elongate your shins out of your ankles. Imagine a small space forming between your shins and your ankles. Relax your ankles.

7. Take the piece of string and elongate your knees out of your shins. Imagine a small space forming between your knees and your shins. Relax your knees.

8. Take the piece of string and elongate your thighs out of your knees. Imagine a small space forming between your thighs and your knees. Relax your thighs.

9. Take the piece of string and elongate your hips out of your thighs. Imagine a small space forming between your hips and your thighs. See how your thigh muscles lengthen. Relax your hips.

10. Take the piece of string and elongate your body out of your hips. Imagine the space between your ribs and your hips lengthening. There is more space for the organs to breathe and relax. Imagine how the space between each rib lengthens.

See the muscles between each rib stretching. Remember to only imagine, avoid trying to move your body upwards or push your chest out. Elongate your torso and think about small spaces forming between each of your ribs, on the left side and on the right side. Relax your abdomen and your chest.

11. Take the piece of string and elongate your neck out of your shoulders, relaxing the shoulders. Imagine a small space forming between your neck and your shoulders. Relax your shoulders.

12. Keeping your chin parallel to the ground, take the piece of string and elongate your head out of your neck. Imagine a small space forming between your head and your neck. See how your neck lengthens towards the sky, while you keep your chin parallel to the ground. See how the space between your ears and your shoulders lengthens. Make sure you imagine the body going upwards, rather than backwards. Feel the release of tension at the back of your neck, as your neck lengthens. Relax your neck.

13. Imagine the piece of string going down your spine, through the middle of each vertebra. Follow the string from the crown of the head, to the top of the spine between your ears. Follow it as it goes down your neck, your upper back, your lower back, all the way down to your tail bone (or coccyx). Now visualise the vertebrae like beads on a string.

14. Keeping your chin parallel to the ground, allow the piece of string to slowly lengthen your spine, softly lifting each vertebrae, pulling the one above away from the one below, one at a time, starting at your tail bone, going up to your lower back, your upper back, your neck and up to the top of the spine between your ears. You can also see your spine as made of rubber and lengthening towards the sky. Your spine and each of the vertebrae are now lengthened and able to breathe and relax. Relax your spine and your back.

15. Now let go of the piece of string and replace it with a balloon hanging above your head. See your body as made of a large piece of rubber. As the balloon floats up, it lengthens the piece of rubber, your body, while the rubber keeps its shape and alignment.

16. Enjoy the feeling for a moment and when you're ready, take a deep breath and open your eyes.

During the visualisation the most common tendencies to avoid are:

- Trying too hard to elongate. This, most often, leads to leaning backwards instead of lengthening. You end up tensing your body rather than relaxing it.
- Lifting the chin and compressing the back of the neck and cervical vertebrae. Instead, keep your chin parallel to the ground and elongate from the crown of your head.
- Puffing the chest out too much and compressing the shoulder blades together. Shoulders should be aligned with the ears when the chin is parallel to the ground, so there is no need to exaggerate by pulling the shoulders back. Shoulders should be relaxed.
- Hips tilting forwards or backwards too much (i.e. spilling water).
- Knees locking as you try to lengthen your body. The body should lengthen with the knees soft.
- Shifting the bodyweight too much on the balls of the feetor placing too much weight on one foot. As you elongate, it is normal to want to shift your body weight forwards, and, if you were running, this would be fine as you'd be using gravity to move forwards. Throughout the day, when you stand in one place, try to check your bodyweight distribution. After you have done this a few times it will only take you 2–3 seconds to scan.

HIP MOVEMENT AND MOBILITY

This is a very important aspect of human movement. The hips provides stability, power and strength to the body.

The way you work with your hips affects the muscles all around your body, directly or indirectly.

Compressing the lumbar spine by tilting your hips forwards, shortens and lengthens specific muscles on the posterior and anterior muscle chain. For example, a forward tilt shortens your hip flexors. Then, when you need your flexors to extend, such as when running, lunging or simply performing a movement that stretches those muscles, they may overstretch and be injured.

This is only one implication of keeping the pelvis tilted forwards. In fact, it impacts every area of the body around it and those areas impact the areas around them. It is all a chain reaction.

There is a lot to write about how a simple position affects several areas, as the body is very interconnected. This book gives you a basic understanding to hopefully make you curious enough to learn more.

Once you adjust your physiology you begin to decompress and reduce the amount of pain and perhaps even eliminate it, if this turns out to be the cause of your pain.

Understanding hip movement and mobility, and how to use it to your advantage is a very important step in physical awareness on your journey to pain-free movement. Further understanding the connection between the lower and upper body through the hips is also critical and you want this connection to be as smooth as possible to ensure that your body functions optimally.

The main connections to be aware of are hip-shoulder, hip-leg and hip-shoulder-arm.

Hip-shoulder connection. As you walk your body moves your hips around an axis (the spine). Your shoulders move in the opposite direction (i.e. right side of the hip moving forwards and left shoulder moving forwards: it's a diagonal connection). Your hips move your shoulders and vice versa. Think the about walking and running movements. Go ahead and move your arms really fast and you will notice your hips move faster and faster, and your legs want to start moving as well.

Hip-leg and hip-shoulder-arm connection. Your hips also move your legs and your shoulders move your arms. But your hips are connected to your shoulders so, by connection, your hips impact the movement of your arms. By the way, that doesn't mean you can't move your arms without the hip movement, but this will cause a greater muscle load on your shoulders and arms. There will always be movement in the hips, even if ever so slightly, because the body is connected like a chain: this is how it was designed to function, as a whole, interconnected unit.

Finally as your arms and legs move, they also move the hands and fingers, feet and toes, respectively. This is all a chain reaction with every area of the body affecting the other.

We can conclude that the hip, when it functions properly, moves the entire body.

When the body moves as it was built to move, in an efficient way: with more output (movement) and less input (stress), this will lighten the load on all the other parts of your body.

Less loading means less muscle tension, which means less pain in the long run. Also, less tension means greater speed. Those of you who are runners looking to get faster, add relaxation to your sprints as well as arm movement. It makes a big difference.

Here's an experiment. If you were to move your arms for a while without moving your hips as well, your arms would get tired much faster than if you also used your hips to move your shoulders and then your arms. It's a chain reaction so if every bit is doing its part, the load spreads to multiple areas, and each area can experience less strain as a result.

Next I want you to understand the terms "tucking" and "clenching in relation to the pelvis, as they are relevant to the exercises later in the book.

Tucking means the bucket of water is tilted backwards, spilling water behind it. Another way to express it is that when you tuck, the belly button looks at the sky. When you tuck, the buttocks push forwards, the lower back rounds and the lumbar spine pushed backwards.

Clenching is when you bring your glutes together, left and right, as opposed to forwards. One of my clients used to say it's as if you're holding a £50 bank note between your buttocks. Hip and lumbar spine movement is minimal but the glutes are tensed.

We will be using this to explain certain movements, particularly the squat. When you squat you don't want to tuck, you want to clench. This engages your glutes and they act as stabilisers for your back. So when you lift a heavy object you use your glutes (and your legs of course) rather than your back.

The tucking (curving the spine backwards) and un-tucking (arching the lumbar spine) exercise is great on its own for mobility. Return to the *Bucket of water* section to practise it. However, attention must be given to and by people who have specific lower back pain (i.e. slipped discs, spine surgery etc.) as this exercise takes the spine through the whole range of motion.

SYNOVIAL FLUID

Synovial fluid is a viscous solution found in the cavities of synovial joints. The principal role of synovial fluid is to reduce friction between the articular cartilages of synovial joints during movement.[8]

Why do you need to know about synovial fluid? Because synovial fluid is to your body what oil is to your car or to the door hinges in your house. When the car parts or door hinges are lubricated, they glide past each other, reducing early damage. There is no impediment to movement and so they last longer.

Synovial fluid does the same thing for your joints, it lubricates them for easy and smooth movement so the cartilages don't grind against each other.

Synovial fluid has the following functions in the body[9]:

1. Lubricates the cartilage at the ends of the bones in the joint.
2. Supplies nutrients to the cartilage.
3. Helps diagnose the cause of joint inflammation in the body in joint diseases like arthritis. The synovium of the joint is the main place where inflammation occurs.

During the warmup before you begin your exercise, you get the synovial fluid lubricating the joints throughout your body. The warmup also raises your heart

---

8 Tamer TM. *Hyaluronan and synovial joint: function, distribution and healing.* Interdisciplinary Toxicology- Available at: www.ncbi.nlm.nih.gov/pmc/articles/.

9 Healthline. *Synovial Fluid Analysis: Purpose, Procedure, and Results.* Available at: www.healthline.com/health/synovial-fluid-analysis.

rate and body temperature and prepares the body for the movements you are about to perform.

It is also important that you take your joints through their full range of motion regularly so that the whole joint is lubricated. Taking joints through their full range of motion will ensure the synovial fluid is present throughout the joint. This is one of the reasons Move Wild is so beneficial. It encompasses movements which take the joints through their full range of motion.

For the lower body, one way to do this is through the full squat we perform at the beginning of each lesson, which you will learn about soon. The full squat takes the ankles, knees and hips through their full range of motion. It also moves, stretches and mobilises the spine, getting it ready for action. The Split Squat, Duck Walk, Frog Jumps and a few others do the same.

Synovial fluid, warmups and the full range of motion are some of the many important aspects of training to ensure the joints stay healthier for longer.

CHAPTER 3. PREPARING FOR MOVE WILD

In this chapter you will simply be introduced to the beginning of your workout. That means warming up and preparing the body for the movements to come.

The warmup ideally raises your heart rate and body temperature and then dynamically stretches the muscles so the risk of injuries is reduced.

With Move Wild exercises, I would argue that the primary movements themselves (i.e. Panther Walk, Crab Walk, Frog jump), performed in a slow, controlled manner and in low repetitions, are a good warmup. However, I am introducing you to forms of warmup you can use in your Move Wild routine, and any routine.

In addition to this warmup, ensure you warmup your wrists, as most Move Wild exercises require wrist mobility. If you perform circular movements with your wrists and stretch them for 2–3 min, it is a good warmup. With the Fluid Movement Stretch, you will have the chance to move your wrists as well...provided you remember.

CARDIOVASCULAR WARMUP

A 10–15 min cardio warmup suffices for the Move Wild session. This is how long you would perform a cardio warmup for almost any workout.

The cardio should begin slowly and gradually increase to around 5–6 intensity on a scale of 1 to 10 (10 being the most intense). This is your own rate of perceived exertion so it's ok to be subjective.

You should breathe a little more heavily at the end of the cardio warmup, but still be able to maintain a conversation.

Depending on your fitness level you could choose the following cardiovascular warmups:

- Running
- Walking
- Brisk walking
- Walking and running
- Cross trainer
- Stair climbing

Once you have done your 10–15 min of cardiovascular warmup you can move on to dynamic stretches.

DYNAMIC STRETCHES

a. Fluid movement stretch

Remember to head to www.movewildacademy.com/move-wild and enter the password "duckwalk" to access all these videos.

The fluid movement stretch looks like The Matrix movements, Tai Chi or Qi Kung for those familiar with the terms. I learnt it from my obstacle course race coach, and it does wonders so I am passing it down to you.

Through the fluid movement stretch, we allow the body to open up by itself, to flow and slowly release the muscles instead of forcing a certain pattern of movement. So take it slowly and be quite comfortable. You might breathe a little faster and attention must be paid to postural hypotension.

Postural hypotension[10] happens when you change positions suddenly, the blood pressure drops fast and you get dizzy. This can happen to anyone, however if you do have blood pressure problems or any health conditions or concerns at all, ensure you talk to your therapist or doctor.

Watch the video where I coach you through the whole exercise on www.move-wildacademy.com/move-wild (password "duckwalk")

---

10 NHS.uk. *Low blood pressure (hypotension)*. Available at: www.nhs.uk/conditions/low-blood-pressure-hypotension/.

Here are a few guidelines to help you with the fluid movement stretch routine:

- Movements are like in the movie the Matrix: slow, long and wide.
- Move your arms and hands in and out from the centre of your body. The hands meet in front of the body around the solar plexus, they push out in opposite directions, go around in a circle and meet back in front of the body to go out again. This is just one way to do it.
- Move your arms at the same time and in symmetry; one goes up, the other down, one left, one right, one in front, one behind etc.
- Perform circular, non-interrupted, fluid movements with your arms and hands. Avoid holding the stretch, jerking, stopping and restarting or changing directions by stopping. Allow the movement to flow in uninterrupted circular paths. As Bruce Lee said: "be as water, my friend". Allow your body to flow naturally. Find your own rhythm.
- Remember to include your neck, wrists and fingers in the stretch sequence as well.
- You torso moves as well, it moves in a circular pattern, side to side and front to back as the arms perform their own circular movements.
- Ensure you include twists, turns and bends of the upper body and allow the lower body to adjust to allow these movements to happen. Don't force anything.
- For the dancer or ice skater in you, think of this movement as a dance. A dance that is slow and looks like a cat stretching after a nap.

There are five levels we usually go through to ensure we stretch every muscle in the body. Remember to warmup your wrists as well.

Level 1: Standing

The circular movements of the arms and trunk and light back bends are performed from a standing position.

Note: every time you bend backwards, try to lengthen up and back so as to avoid compressing the lower back. In this way you elongate from the top of your head upwards and backwards, using the piece of string you already know about.

You will feel the sides of your body stretching, as well as all around your shoulders.

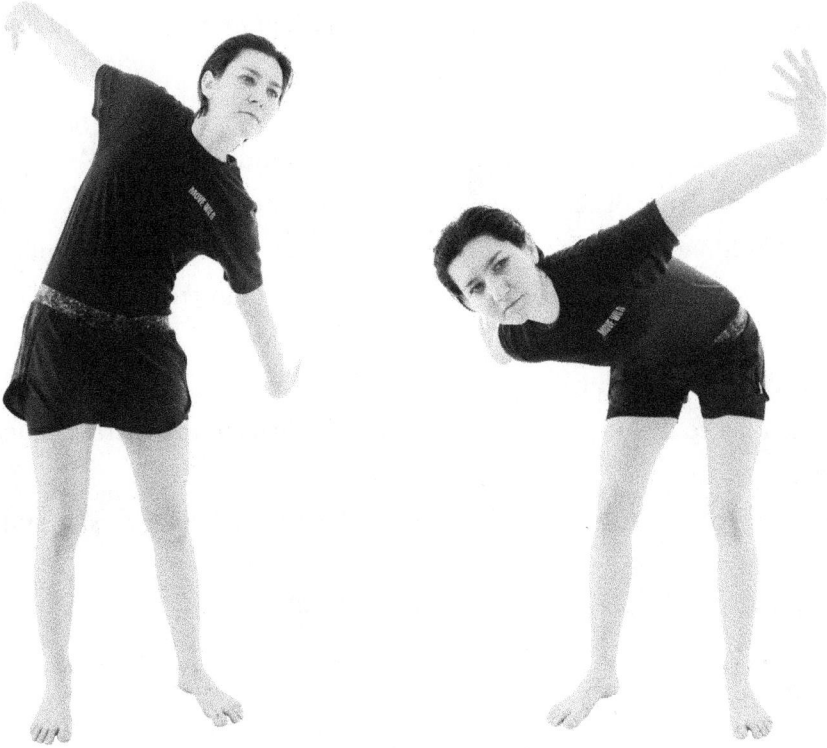

Fluid Movement Stretch, standing

Level 2: High side lunge

Step to one side and bend the knee, while keeping the other leg straight. Repeat the same arm and body movements, even slower than before. In this position you begin to open the hips and slowly stretch your hip flexors, while still stretching the trunk and shoulders. Reach as far as you can in every direction.

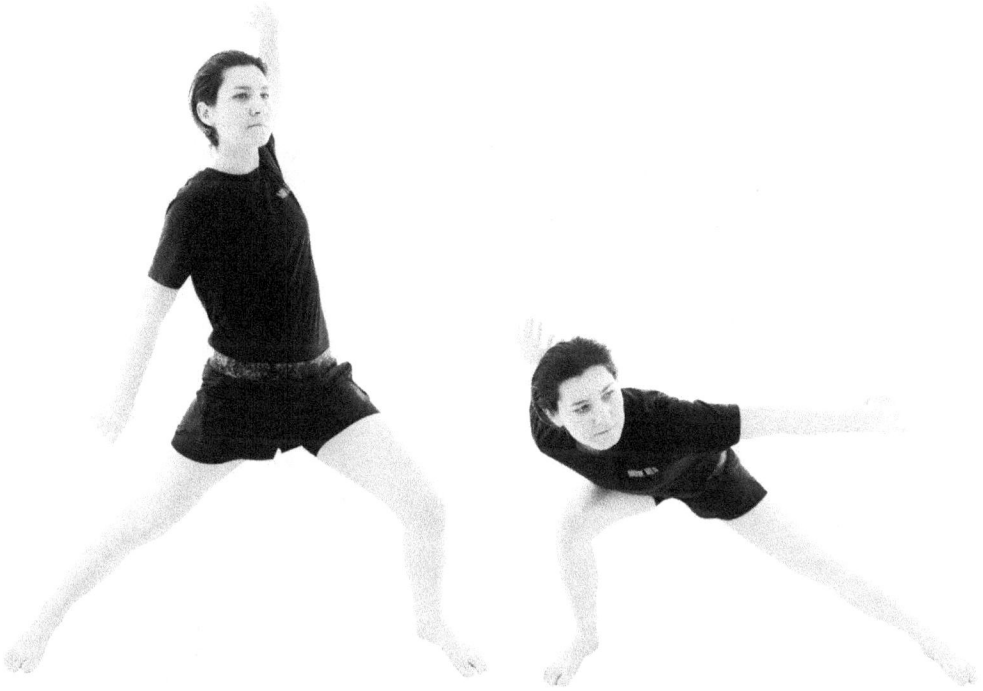

Fluid Movement Stretch, high side lunge

Level 3: Front lunge

At this stage you can try deeper back bends, remembering to elongate upwards and backwards, and just as in swimming, open up with both arms, starting from the front of your hips and stretching your arms as far back as you can.

Keep moving the arms in circular, uninterrupted patterns. Followed by a counter stretch forwards and side bends (arms come up and over the head) on each side.

Go deeper into the hip flexors. Don't force anything, just let the body naturally release. You don't need to stay in this position for too long and if you are having trouble with balance, move the front foot to the side to create more space between your legs. If you're still struggling place the back heel on the floor as well.

45

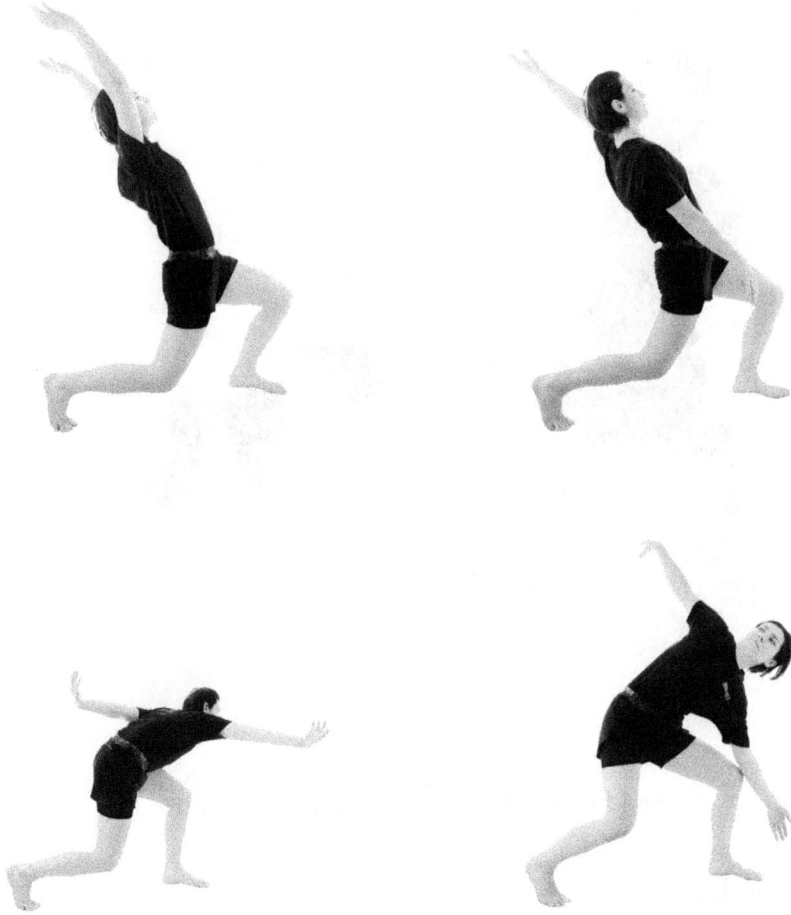

Fluid Movement Stretch, front lunge

Level 4: Low side lunge

This is similar to the high side lunge but go further to the side and lower, keeping both feet and heels on the ground, and point your toes on both feet forwards.

You should now feel a stretch in your adductors, inside the thigh, as well as the glutes on the side with the bent leg if they are very tight.

Until now you have focused more on hip extension. This and the next stretch move from extension focus to flexion focus on the bent leg. You will, however, have hip extension on the extended leg.

Whilst I'm directing your attention to certain areas of your body, nothing actually moves in isolation. Throughout the book, each exercise has a focus area, or a few areas, but the body works as a whole.

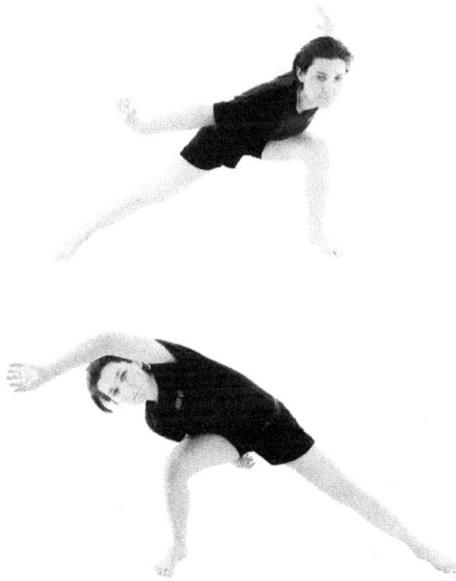

Fluid Movement Stretch, low side lunge

Level 5: Low side stretch

Bend one leg under your hips with the heel off the ground. Extend the other leg straight to the side with toes up, forming a 90 degree angle at the groin. Repeat the same upper body movements as before, but now you are also challenging your balance skills, unless you choose to place your hand on the floor.

You will feel a stretch at the back of the stretched-out leg.

If you struggle to get into this position, stand with your feet hip width apart and crouch. Let your heel come off the floor. Then extend one leg to the side and you are in position.

If your muscles are very tight and painful, skip this level. As you practise this stretch regularly, you'll be able to go all the way down.

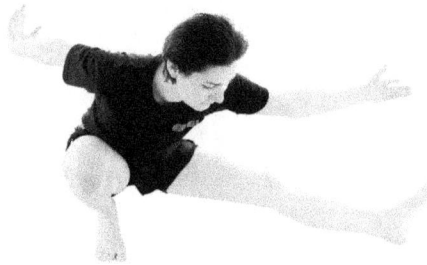

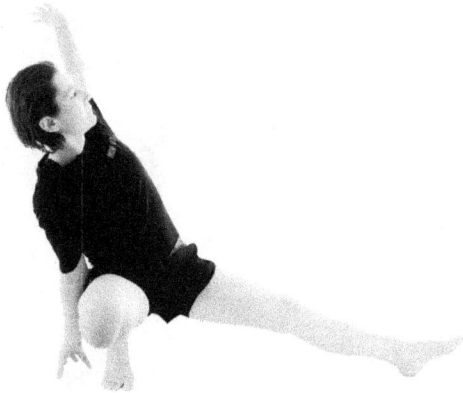

Fluid Movement Stretch, low side stretch

b. Fascia stretches

You can also use the following dynamic stretches. I called them fascia stretches for the purposes of the book but the fluid movement stretch shown above also stretches the fascia.

This warmup sequence stretches and mobilises almost every facet of the body: front, back and sides. It roughly follows the lines of the fascia.

The fascia is "a thin layer of connective tissue covering, supporting, or connecting the muscles or inner organs of the body"[11]. It "surrounds and holds every organ, blood vessel, bone, nerve fibre and muscle in place"[12].

Movement stretches the fascia, while lack of movement may thicken and tighten it. That's when it begins to restrict further movement and can reduce mobility and enable painful knots to develop[13]. This is why movement is so important and poor movement is one of the causes of pain and lack of mobility in our bodies.

This routine is appropriate for those who find the Fluid Movement Stretch challenging. Of course you can perform both stretch routines if you wish. Fascia stretches could be useful for older people, or those of you who find general mobility and flexibility challenging. It could also be an alternative option for those who suffer from non-specific low back pain (i.e. not from a slipped disc, accident or surgery).

There are three planes of movement we all go through.

1. Sagittal: moving forwards and backwards
2. Frontal: moving side to side
3. Transverse: rotation

Fascia stretches go through each plane of movement and mobilise and stretch almost every area of the body.

For each plane, the upper body performs the same movement sequence while the lower body changes from standing to stepping forwards and back and then to a little hop forwards and back.

Due to the up and down movement, you might feel light-headed from hypotension. Ensure you move in a slow and controlled way, there is no need to rush.

---

11 Collinsdictionary.com. *Fascia definition and meaning | Collins English Dictionary*. Available at: https://www.collinsdictionary.com/dictionary/english/fascia

12 Johns Hopkins Medicine. *Muscle Pain: It May Actually Be Your Fascia*. Available at: www.hopkinsmedicine.org/health/wellness-and-prevention/muscle-pain-it-may-actually-be-your-fascia.

13 Johns Hopkins Medicine. Muscle Pain: It May Actually Be Your Fascia. Available at: www.hopkinsmedicine.org/health/wellness-and-prevention/muscle-pain-it-may-actually-be-your-fascia.

Ensure you warmup your wrists in preparation for Move Wild floor exercises as well.

Sagittal plane

The sagittal plane divides the body into left and right sides. In this instance the movement is forwards and backwards.

Standing

Step forwards with the right foot and bend over to reach the front toes (bend knees as needed), allowing the back to curl. Then stand back up again.

Repeat 10 reps with the right foot forwards and 10 reps with the left foot forwards. I am giving you a guideline of how many to execute, but you can break the sets down as you wish. It is not about how many reps you do, but to execute the exercise with the correct form and warmup properly. As a guideline, 7-10 reps is a good number for your joints to be ready for the next movements.

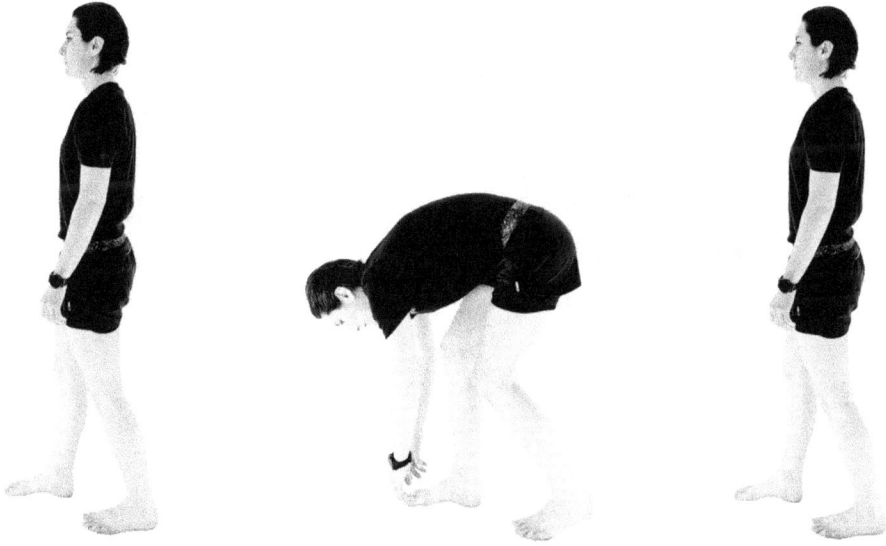

Fascia stretch, sagittal plane, standing

Stepping

Carry out the same movement but this time bring the right foot back next to the left after each repetition. Then step out again with the right foot and repeat.

Count 10 reps with the right foot and 10 reps with the left foot.

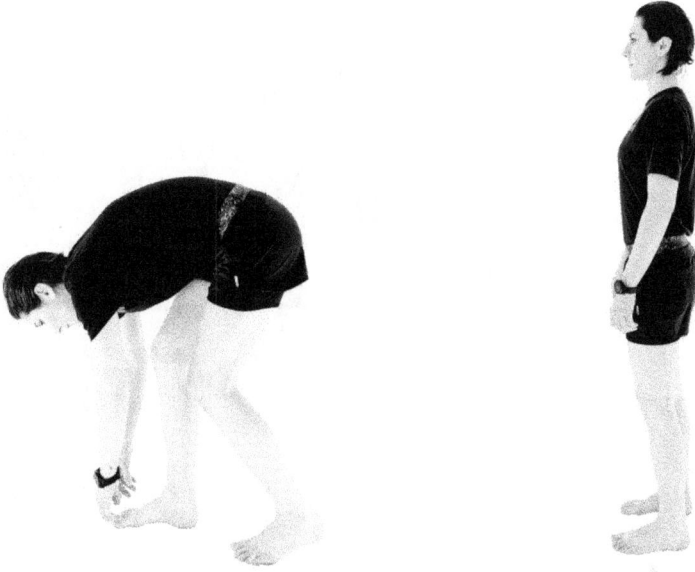

Fascia stretch, sagittal plane, stepping

Hopping

The same movement but this time with a little hop when stepping out with the leading foot. Keep the back foot off the floor when you bend forwards. This challenges your balance. However, if you have trouble with balance, do the hop and place the back foot on the floor. Once you have touched the floor, hop back to the start position.

Complete 10 reps on the right and 10 reps on the left.

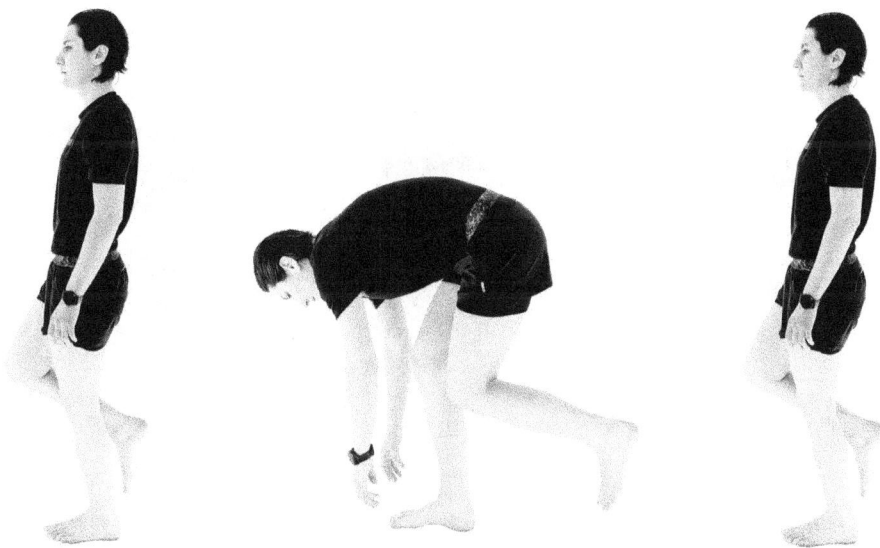

Fascia stretch, sagittal plane, hopping

Frontal plane – outside movement

The frontal plane divides the body into front and back. Movement will be to the side and in this case on the side of the leg that steps forwards.

If this gets too complicated head to www.movewildacademy.com/move-wild and enter the password "duckwalk" to access all the videos for more instructions. Search for the fascia stretched in the warmup section.

Standing

Step forwards with the right foot, bend your torso to the right side (towards the outside of the front leg) and lift the left arm up and over your head, towards the right side.

As the body straightens hold the right foot on the spot and repeat with the same foot forwards for 10 reps. Then place the left foot forwards and do the same movement towards the same side (right side).

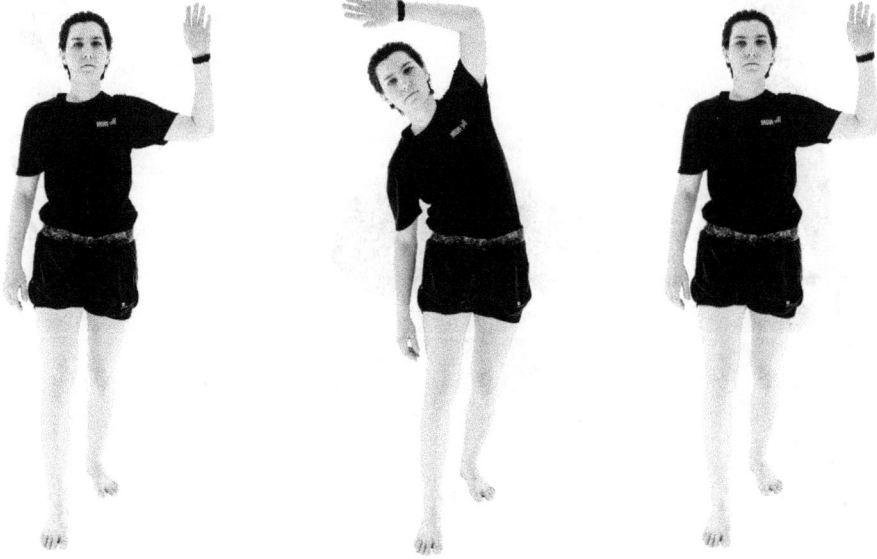

Fascia stretch, frontal, outside movement, standing

Stepping

Carry out the same movement but this time bring the right foot back next to the left after each repetition. Then step out again with the right foot and repeat.

Complete 10 reps with the right foot forward, still bending from your waist towards the right side.

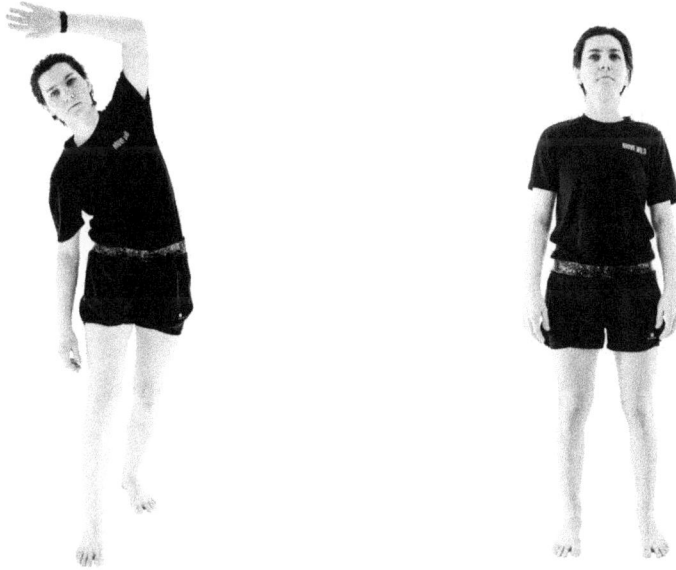

Fascia stretch, frontal, outside movement, stepping

Then, while bending to the same side, step with the left foot forward and repeat the same movement for another 10 reps.

Hopping

Execute the same movement with a little hop when stepping out with the leading foot. As before, try to balance on the front foot and keep the back foot off the floor. Then hop back to the start position. Keep bending towards the right side for 10 reps and then just change the leading foot and carry on for another 10 reps.

Frontal plane – inside movement

Now we move on to the left side. This is the same movement, with the right foot forward and then the left, but bending to the left side instead of the right.

You will go through standing, stepping and hopping with the right and then the left foot forwards while bending from the waist towards the left at all times.

Transverse plane

The final plane is the transverse, where we twist the body. Here the body is divided into top (above the hips) and bottom (below the hips). By now you know the stages of standing, stepping and hopping. We will do the same again now.

Standing

Step forwards with the right foot and reach towards the bottom of the back foot, as if you want to pick up a rock off the floor behind you.

Pick up the rock, stand up and swing both arms over the opposite right shoulder, as if you want to throw the rock over your shoulder. Allow the body to twist naturally as much it as feels comfortable, controlling the movement.

Hold the right foot on the spot as you execute the same sequence for 10 reps.

When you change to left foot forwards you pick up the rock from the back foot, which is the right foot now, and throw it over your left shoulder. Repeat for 10 reps on this side as well.

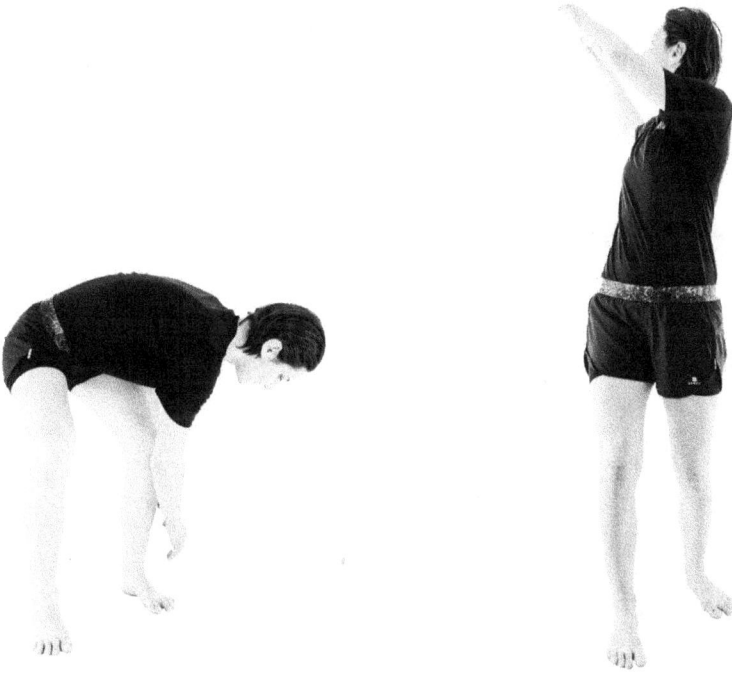

Fascia stretch, transverse, standing

Stepping

Complete the same exercise but this time you step out with the leading foot and step back to standing position, as you have done in the frontal and sagittal planes.

Perform 10 reps with the right foot forwards and 10 reps with the left foot forwards.

Hopping

The last 2 sets of 10 reps are with the hop you are hopefully used to by now. Remember to try and balance on the front foot.

Complete the same movement on the left and right sides with the hop forwards and hop back between each repetition.

Note:

I recommend you maintain the sagittal, frontal and then transverse plane order, and keep the standing, stepping, hopping order as well.

You want to begin with the more simple movements and gradually build up to the more complex ones such as twists. I ordered them this way for this reason.

The simplest movement in the sequence is the sagittal standing, thus is it our first exercise.

The frontal plane, where you go left and right, is easier to play with. For example you can keep the same foot forwards and bend left and then right, you can order the inside/outside sequence as you wish, but I recommend to keep the standing, stepping, hopping order.

Remember: go from simple to complex.

CHAPTER 4. MOVE WILD EXERCISES

For the purpose of teaching the Move Wild exercises are grouped in three main categories:

1. Strength
2. Balance and body weight transfer
3. Flexibility

Although they are grouped in these categories they are not set in stone. All strength exercises have an element of balance and flexibility, although they might be predominantly perceived as body weight strength exercises.

With this in mind let's go through the exercises in the first category, strength. And remember to head to www.movewildacademy.com/move-wild and enter the password "duckwalk" to access all these videos and more.

STRENGTH

There are 15 different types of exercise aimed at building strength, coordination and agility. However they also develop balance, mobility and flexibility. From these 15 fundamental strength exercises, variations can be derived.

1. Full Squat
2. Panther Walk
3. Crab Walk
4. Frog Jump Spot
5. Frog Jump Forwards
6. Frog Jump Side

7. Frog Jump Twisted
8. Frog Leap
9. Tiger Walk
10. Crocodile Stalk
11. Duck Walk
12. Split Squat
13. Cross Frog
14. Side Monkey
15. Bunny Hop

FULL SQUAT

Benefits

It strengthens major stability muscles – quadriceps, gluteus maximus, hamstrings, core muscles, as well as smaller joint stability muscles – feet, toes, ankles, knees, hips.

It also strengthens foot arches which then helps with over pronation and certain foot, ankle and knee injuries. Your feet are your foundation. Everything begins from the roots. Weak stability muscles contribute to injuries. The full squat helps to create strong foundations. It's one of the most natural human movements.

It mobilises your ankles, knees and hips as well stretching the back and glutes and it takes the joints through their full range of motion ensuring complete joint mobility.

Technical points

With your feet about hip width apart, toes facing forwards and the tripod firmly rooted on the ground, align and elongate your body. Activate your abdominal muscles and keep your chest out and proud throughout the movement.

Bend your knees without lifting the heels off the ground or taking the weight off the heels.

When you feel you can't bend your knees anymore while keeping the weight on the heels, take your hips back and sit down as if you want to sit on a small nursery chair right underneath you.

Look ahead at all times and try to keep the toes facing forwards, while the knees track your feet (i.e. they don't buckle in or push out to the side). Once you are sitting down in the squat, try to elongate your body and relax your shoulders.

If you struggle to keep your balance, stretching out the hands in front serves as counterbalance.

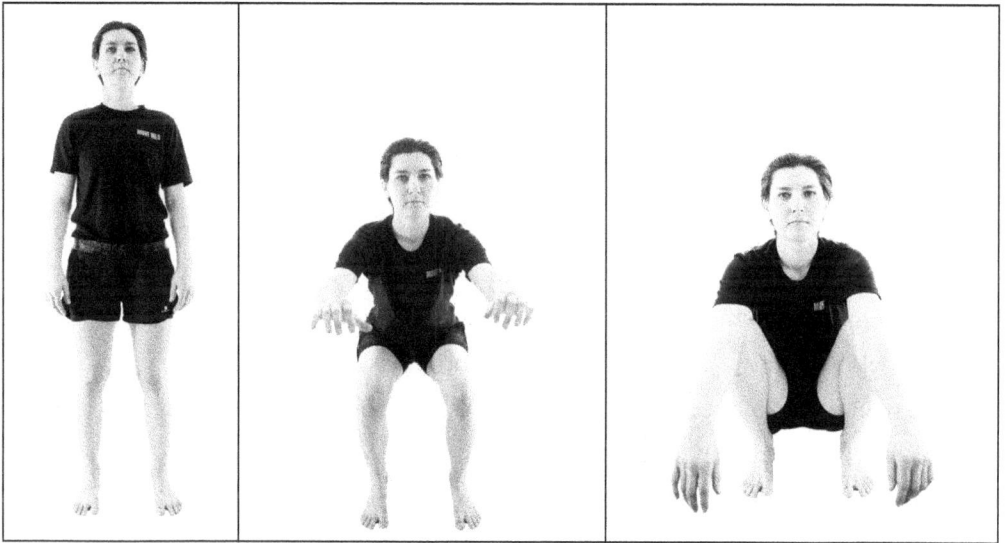

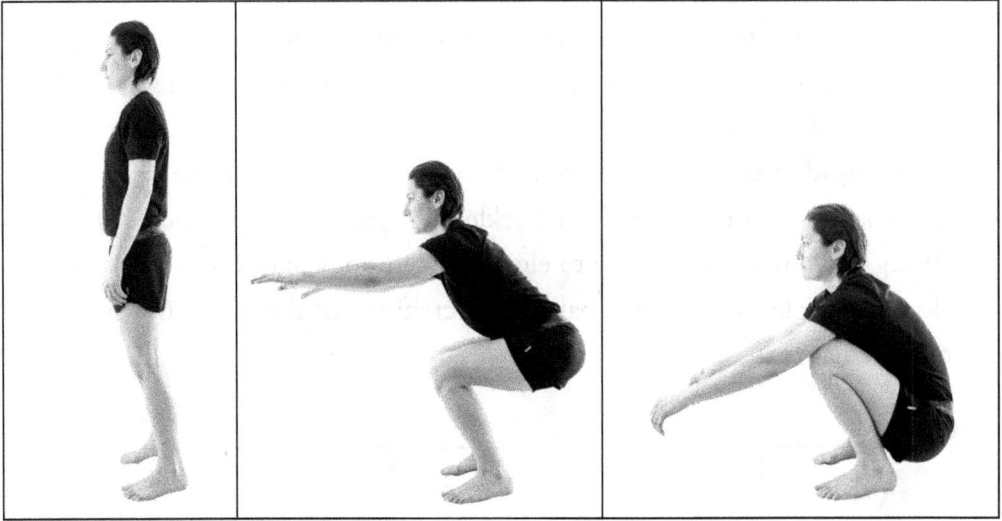

Full Squat, squatting down

When you stand up it is important to still keep your chest proud and abdominal muscles tensed. The movement is the opposite of going down, the same level of control. Below there are a few points to remember when you stand up from the squat.

Lift the upper body first, not you buttocks. As strange as it sounds, the buttocks are underneath all the time, they do not lift first.

Look ahead, but without lifting your chin. Elongate your body, drop your shoulders, lift your chest and look ahead as you stand back up, pushing through the tripod.

About half-way up, clench (do not tuck) your buttocks. Imagine it's like a platform lifting you up from underneath together with the hamstrings.

Stand up with a slow, controlled and uninterrupted movement (see *Full Squat, standing up*). When you move slowly, you recruit all the muscles; this makes the exercise more challenging and addresses many imbalances and weaknesses in the body.

Why do you need to activate your buttocks you ask? One good reason is to get the body to fire up these very important stabiliser muscles. These muscles play an important part in preventing injuries such as to the lower back and knees when we walk, run, push, pull, carry, lift and so on. The glutes are big muscles with an important role, thus they need to fire and do their job for the benefit of the whole body.

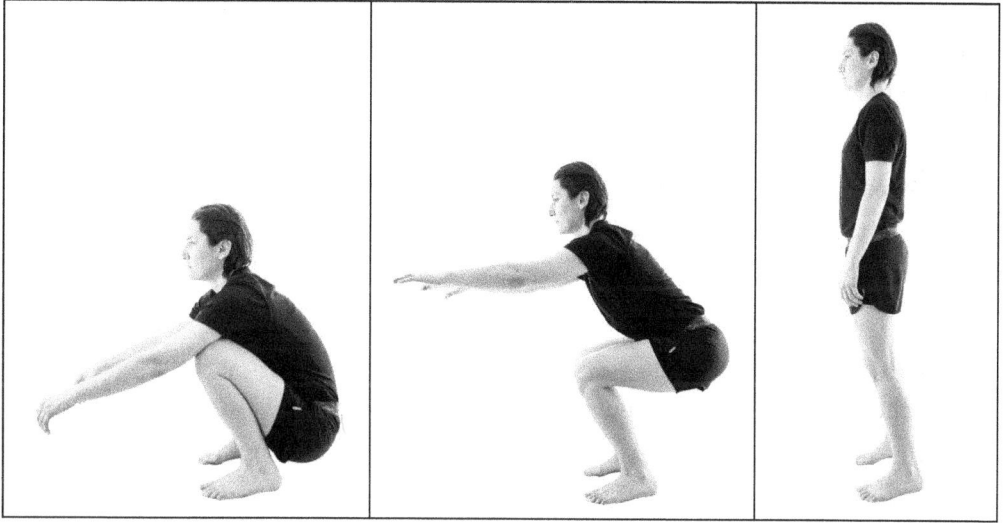

Full Squat, standing up

A few more tips:

Breathe out on the way down and on the way up, and breathe in when you are in the final positions (standing and squatting).

Breathing out makes your belly button go inwards towards your spine (if you breathe correctly) and your abdominal muscles activate, which is what you want when you make an effort.

If your heels come off the ground place a wedge underneath them such as a stick or a thin book. As your ankles and hips mobilize and strengthen you will not need them anymore. You can also use an incline with your toes going down the slope. Avoid high wedges or steep slopes though, as it can overload the knees. You also want to make it somewhat challenging so a steep slope won't benefit you.

When standing on an incline or using a wedge, pay close attention to body weight distribution. Do not shift your body weight away from the heels and onto the toes as that overloads the knees. Hold the pressure on the heels as you go up and down.

With my clients I use a stick to point out how the hips move in between the shoulders and the knees by engaging the glutes. It actually helps them to understand how the body should move. This is a more advanced way of looking at the squat so don't worry if you don't get it. Make sure you visit the Move Wild videos to learn more.

Take a stick and break it into two pieces. Where the stick breaks are the hips. The top of the stick is the head and shoulders and the bottom of the stick is the knees and ankles.

When standing up the hips should move forwards, in between the shoulders and the knees.

The head, shoulders and knees shouldn't move backwards too much when you stand up, until the end. The hips lift everything up by wedging in between.

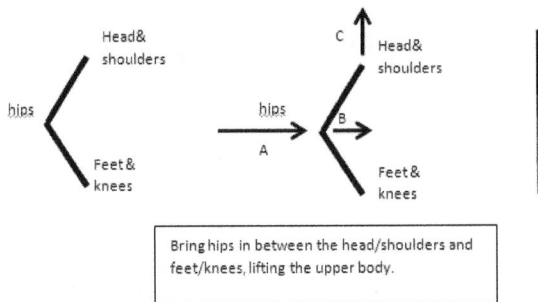

The Stick Example

Common errors and/or weaknesses to be aware of:

- Jerky movements and loss of balance. This may indicate muscle weakness at some point in the movement. These are most obvious when, at the bottom of the squat, there is a sudden drop or on the way up until about half-way it looks and feels like you cannot control the movement.
- Knees buckling or pushing out excessively and out of alignment.

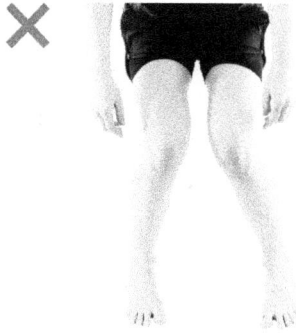

Full Squat, knees buckling

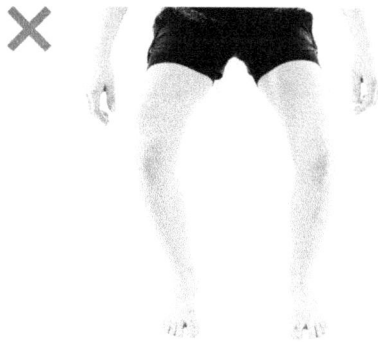

Full Squat, knees pushing out

- Placing more body weight on one leg than the other. This may indicate a weakness or injury on the side with less weight. It can be an injury, muscles weakness and/or tightness, and shifting the body weight may indicate protection for the side.
- Slouching and rounding the back. Always keep your chest proud and core tensed.
- Buttocks are tucked in instead of clenched, which rounds the lower back and causes the shoulders to round forwards as well. Buttocks should clench, not tuck. *Full Squat, tucked buttocks* shows a rather extreme example of this to give a clear imagine of how the back rounds when the buttocks tuck instead of clenching.

65

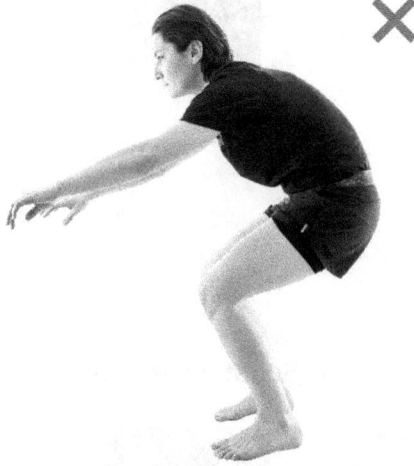

Full Squat, tucked buttocks

- Buttocks come up first when standing up, knees straighten before hips come forwards (see *Full squat, buttocks lift first*). This could mean the glutes are not activated properly on the way up. The torso should lead the movement with chest proud.

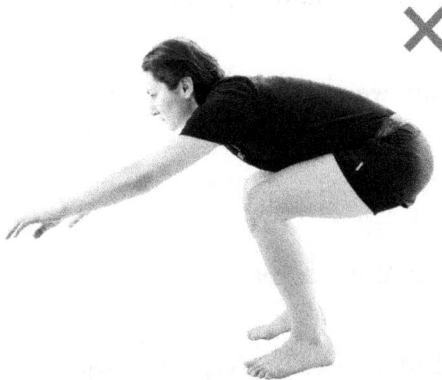

Full squat, buttocks lift first

- On the way down into the squat, sticking the buttocks out before bending the knees at all. Ensure the knees bend first, while keeping the heels on the ground and weight on the tripods. The idea is to squat as if sitting on a small nursery chair placed right behind the heels. You wouldn't stick your butt out without

66

bending your knees to sit down, would you? You would have the chair under you and you'd sit almost straight down.

- Lifting the heels or the toes off the ground at any point throughout the movement. The tripod should be firmly rooted on the ground at all times.
- Shifting the body weight onto the toes too much. In this case you can think about shifting just 51% of the body weight onto the heels and it normally rebalances the weight distribution.
- Pushing on the toes when standing up instead of pushing or standing up through the heels. This is peculiar to individuals who cannot or do not know how to recruit the gluteus muscles. In this case you can perform the squat higher to help form the correct body awareness and bodyweight distribution and gradually strengthen the muscles which need to be used. This should help redistribute the body weight and help you activate the correct muscles.
- Looking down. As a general rule, the body follows the head and the head follows the eyes; where the eyes go the body follows. Ideally the back of your neck should be straight at all times.
- Lifting the chin when standing up. The chest should be proud and the chin should stay in the same position relative to the chest; when standing up the chin is parallel to the ground.
- Toes pointing out and/or knees pushing out excessively or buckling. For the purpose of developing a good alignment and body awareness ensure that your toes point forwards and the knees track the feet, pointing neither inwards nor outwards. This way pronation (foot rolls inwards excessively) and supination (foot rolls outwards excessively) are minimised. Ensure that feet are hip width apart, if possible.

Toes pointing out	Supination	Toes pointing forward
✕	✕	✓

Full Squat, incorrect and correct foot position

- Shoulders shrugging. Remember to relax your shoulders and make space between the ears and the shoulders.

PANTHER WALK

Benefits

The Panther Walk is a fabulous upper body exercise which strengthens the shoulder muscles all around while also mobilising and stabilising. It's a good comeback exercise after a shoulder injury to gradually build the strength back up.

It tones and strengthens the arms, legs and core muscles: abdominal muscles, back, pelvis, diaphragm. The core muscles are responsible for posture so you want the all-round muscle strength and stability. What is most important is that this exercise also works on the inner core muscles. These are the deep stability muscles, not your six pack, and they're more important than that as they support the spine and overall posture.

The Panther Walk also mobilises and strengthens the stability muscles in your feet, ankles, knees and hips for better balance, mobility, control and general movement, reducing risk of injury (including repetitive stress injuries in the wrists) in the long run.

An overlooked benefit for fitness and movement is the fact that you actually stretch and strengthen the soles of the feet, toes and Achilles tendon, especially when this is performed barefoot. Normally we look to train the muscles we see and feel, the ones that look good. However it's often the overlooked areas of your body which give you problems, isn't it? That pain you feel in the sole of your foot for example.

Let's take a look at how to perform the Panther Walk.

Technical points

Begin with the feet hip width apart, lower yourself into a full squat, rock onto your toes and place your hands and knees on the ground. Wrists are under the shoulders, knees under the hips and the back is in neutral position – that is with the natural spinal curves.

From there, activate your core and lift your knees a few cm off the floor, while making sure you keep your weight distributed evenly on both feet and hands.

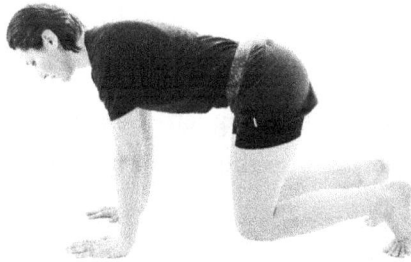

Panther Walk, start position

To move, place your left hand forwards and your right foot forwards slightly. Begin walking in a hand-and-opposite-foot sequence (i.e. left hand, right foot, right hand, left foot...) while keeping the knees bent and as close to the floor as possible. Knees move straight forwards beneath your body and not out to the side.

69

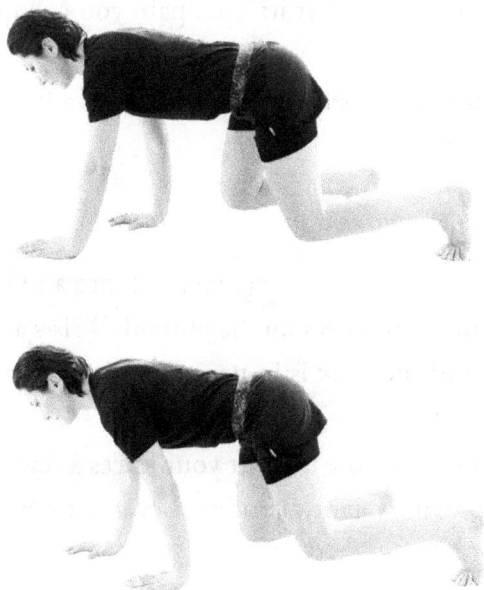

Panther Walk: walking forwards

Try to keep hips low and stable, avoiding left-right hip movement. To achieve this you should use your core to stabilise the position instead of transferring the body weight from one side to the other.

Your spine should be in neutral alignment throughout.

Avoid lifting your hips in the air. If you end up with your hips in the air, stop, reset and try again. Perform the exercise only as long as you can keep the form.

To move forwards, shift your body weight onto your arms, rather than pushing against the ground with your feet – this is movement through bodyweight transfer.

Take very small strides with your feet and look ahead, just in front of your hands, rather than at your knees.

Aim for a fluid, uninterrupted movement, placing your hands and feet softly on the ground as if you want to test the ground before putting your whole bodyweight on it. Stabilise your shoulders and shoulder blades and engage your latissimus dorsi muscles (the large, flat muscle on the back which stretches to the sides, under and behind the arm). This way you teach your body to fire particular muscle groups to perform the movement.

As your hands lift off the floor, relax you arms and allow the shoulders to rotate freely in the shoulder sockets. There is no need to stay tensed all the time. Learn to activate and relax your muscles when it's appropriate.

Imagine you are a panther out hunting and breathe as you normally would, a continuous breathing pattern.

Common errors and/or weaknesses to be aware of:

- Placing more body weight on the arms or the legs – this could be an indication of weakness in the upper or lower body. It is common to use the legs more as they are stronger.
- Lifting the hips and knees high above the ground. Your core muscles don't work as much. It's as if you perform press-ups with your hips in the air. There is a variation of press-ups where the hips are in the air but that's not what you are trying to do here.

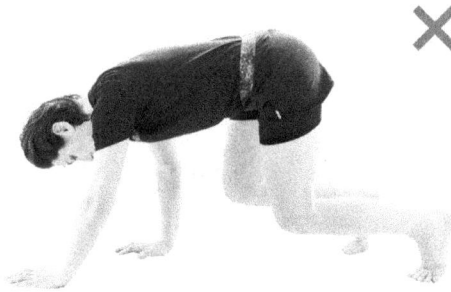

Panther Walk, hips too high

- Tilting hips from side to side when walking. This could indicate weak core strength and poor stability. The core should brace in order to keep the body from swaying side to side and the hips should be as stable as possible.
- Knees going out to the side. Although this can be a variation of the Panther Walk, in this case the knees should move forwards right under the body.
- The stride is too long ending up with the knees under the chest. This will lift the hips. However, if you have the body awareness and strength to stay very low, this can be a variation of the original movement.

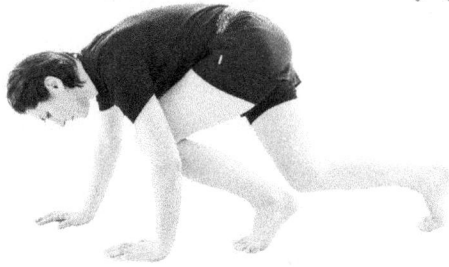

Panther Walk, stride too long

- The stride is too short and you end up stretched out too much. When learning, the knees should stop roughly under the hips. Later, as the body strengthens, you can shorten or lengthen the strides to create variations and make the movement more challenging.
- Looking at the knees and lifting the hips or looking too far forwards and compressing the cervical spine. The neck should be straight, eyes looking just in front of the hands.

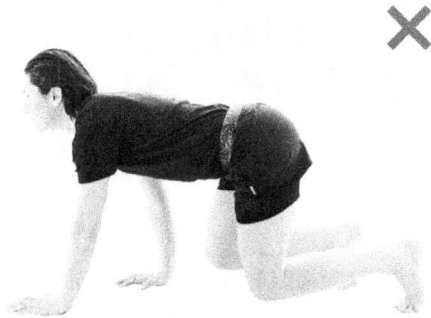

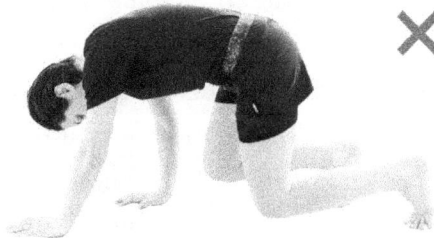

Panther Walk: incorrect neck positions

- Sinking into the shoulders or bringing the shoulder blades tightly together. There is no need for either. Deltoids, core and lats must be activated to stabilise the shoulders and the back should be straight across the shoulders as well as from top to bottom.
- Straightening the knees when walking. Try to keep the knees very close to the ground (without touching) at all times. Don't stretch out the back leg; there is no need. Take strides just as much as you need to bring the knee under the hip while keeping your core tight and your shoulders braced. Think of the movement as coming from your core. I like to say you should "move with your core".

Note:

You can perform the Panther Walk forwards and backwards. You can also find variations on the original movement such as moving in "hand-same foot sequence" or with knees pointing out to the side or bringing the knees further forwards than your hips once you have that body awareness.

Panther Walk backwards

The same points apply as for the Panther Walk forwards. The difference is that you will have to be a lot more compact to avoid stretching out to much and pushing off with your hands.

You actually want to gracefully transfer your bodyweight on to your legs and lift your hands off the ground softly and in a controlled way.

Walking backwards, you should take even smaller steps with your feet, while the arms take longer strides travelling all the way in front of your knees. You still keep the hand-opposite leg sequence.

A great tip is to look behind through your legs to see where you're going.

Progressions:

- Place a tennis ball on the lower back and try to walk without dropping the ball.
- Walk uphill and, especially, downhill.
- Learn variations from our website.

You can go towww.movewildacademy.com/move-wild and enter the password "duck-walk" to access all the videos for more instructions. Videos are also easier to follow.

CRAB WALK

Benefits

The Crab Walk is another great exercise to tone up the upper body, particularly triceps, and stabilise and mobilise the shoulder joint. Some therapists use this exercise with clients who had shoulder injuries to improve strength, stability and mobility in the joint.

It also opens up the chest and improves overall posture, when executed correctly.

It can strengthen the core and stability muscles in your feet, ankles, knees and hips for better balance, stability, control and general movement, reducing the risk of injury.

Let's not forget the overlooked areas of the body such as the wrists and ankles, for which this exercise is excellent.

Technical points

We will begin from a standing position, with the feet hip width apart. You then lower yourself into a full squat and place your hands on the ground behind you. Point your fingers in the same direction as your toes, forwards.

Your body is facing upwards (supine) with your weight is evenly distributed between the 4 limbs.

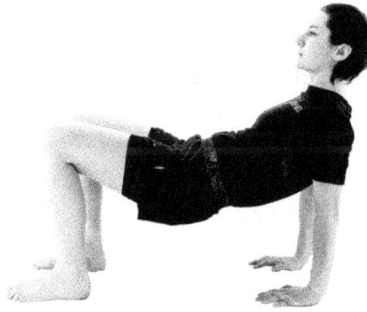

Crab Walk: start position

Tense your core, lift your hips up as high as you can and lengthen your neck out of your shoulders (not lifting your chin, but lengthening from the crown), or think about lowering your shoulders as a shoulder shrug down rather than up. This activates the latissimus dorsi muscles and stabilises the shoulder joint.

You have yet to move but you are in the best starting position. Take your time to feel and remember this stance. You can just hold the position and then relax and hold it up again. You don't need to move until you are ready.

When you are ready, simply take a step with your right foot, placing the ball of your foot on the ground first, then the heel, and the opposite hand. To move you first need to shift the body weight; if there is weight on a limb, you cannot lift and move it without falling or making jerky movements.

As with the Panther Walk you are moving in a foot-opposite-hand sequence; right foot, left hand, left foot, right hand.

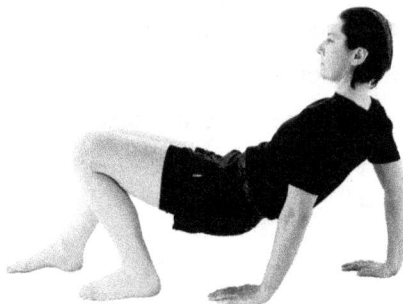

Crab Walk: walking forwards

Some of my clients find this movement challenging at the beginning. This is absolutely fine. If you can't lift your feet or hands off the floor, begin by just holding the position for a set time, let's say 1 min, then relax for 30 sec, then hold again for 1 min. Perform this for 3–4 sets of 3–5 repetitions each.

Continue doing this until you can lift one hand off the floor. It might take days or weeks. Have patience, it will happen. Once you can lift your hands off the floor, you don't need to move. Instead there is another stage you can go on to. You can just lift one hand at a time a few centimetres off the floor, hold it for a set amount of time, let's say 5 sec, then put it back down and try with the other hand. Perform these as many times as you can but no more if your form begins to alter.

If you can lift one hand and not the other, don't worry. Continue trying you lift it until both arms get strong enough to support the weight alone. You can also go back to just holding the position if you prefer.

Remember one important thing: patience is key to learning any Move Wild complex movement.

Allow your shoulders to freely rotate in their sockets as the hands move forwards, relaxing from the shoulder every time you lift the hand off the ground. Place your hands and feet gently on the ground.

Movement should be soft and fluid. This is achieved through efficient body weight distribution and bodyweight transfer.

Common errors and/or weaknesses to be aware of:

- Sinking the head into the shoulders. It looks like the space between the ears and the shoulders is smaller. Use the piece of string you have already learnt about to elongate and lift the neck and head out of the shoulders or think about lengthening the space between the ears and the shoulders. You can also think about lowering the shoulders.

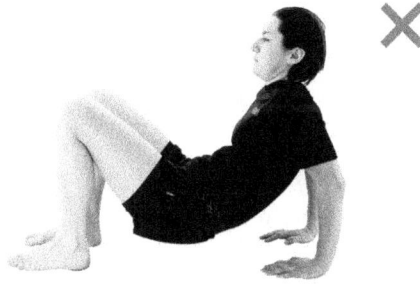

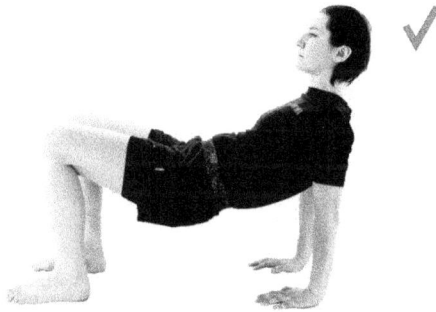

Crab Walk, incorrect and correct head position

- Everything else is good but the hips are very low. The hips should be as high as you can make them whilst keeping all the other elements of the form. Try to keep the hips no lower than mid-height at all times.
- Stepping with the heels and/or not placing the toes down before taking the next step. This keeps the body weight on the arms and makes the movement inefficient; you should step with your toes first which helps mobilise the ankle joint. It's not incorrect to step with your heels, but it helps to get that movement in the joint. However you do want to place your toes on the floor so that the feet take on their share of the bodyweight.
- Fingers not pointing the same way as the toes. This is common as the wrists can feel very painful. We don't stretch the wrists and forearms as much as other parts of the body and the position is especially painful on the inside of the wrist. In this case point your fingers in a direction with which you feel comfortable until they mobilise and strengthen and then slowly guide them

to the desired end position, facing the same way as the toes. When the fingers point a different way there is also less shoulder stability.

Notes:

When going uphill tense and use the hamstrings to pull your body forwards or up inclines. Use them as biceps.

You can perform the Crab Walk forwards, backwards or to the side.

FROG JUMP SPOT

Benefits

The Frog Jump, any version of it, is an excellent exercise to work out your quads, your upper body and core. When it is performed with control, your core does most of the job.

It also strengthens, stretches and mobilises wrists, hips, back, knees and ankles. These joints, particularly wrists, knees and ankles, can do with stronger stability muscles, and the Frog Jump offers just that, improving your balance, stability, control and general movement.

The glutes and adductors (inner thigh) in particular benefit from stretching. The frog jump is a great hip opener and mobilises the area, which in turn reduces the frequency and severity of pain.

Technical points

As we do with all exercises, we begin by squatting. Place your feet hip width apart, lower yourself into a Full Squat, rock onto your toes, point the knees outwards and place your hands on the ground in front of you, as in the *Frog Jump Spot*.

The hands are at a comfortable distance from your body, and you don't need to transfer your body weight forwards at all. If your body moves forwards your hands are placed too far in front of you. So place your hands as far as you can without shifting your bodyweight.

Hold your feet under your hips with the knees pointing out.

When you're ready to execute the exercise, shift your body weight onto your arms until your shoulders are aligned with your wrists. Avoid resting your knees on your elbows.

Lock in (tense) your abdominal muscles and gently and with the greatest control lift your feet off the ground. Although it is called a frog "jump", you want to avoid jumping as this movement is not controlled. So lift as opposed to pushing against the ground or jumping.

Land back on the same spot by placing your feet softly down on the floor, as opposed to dropping back on the ground without control, as you would if you jumped.

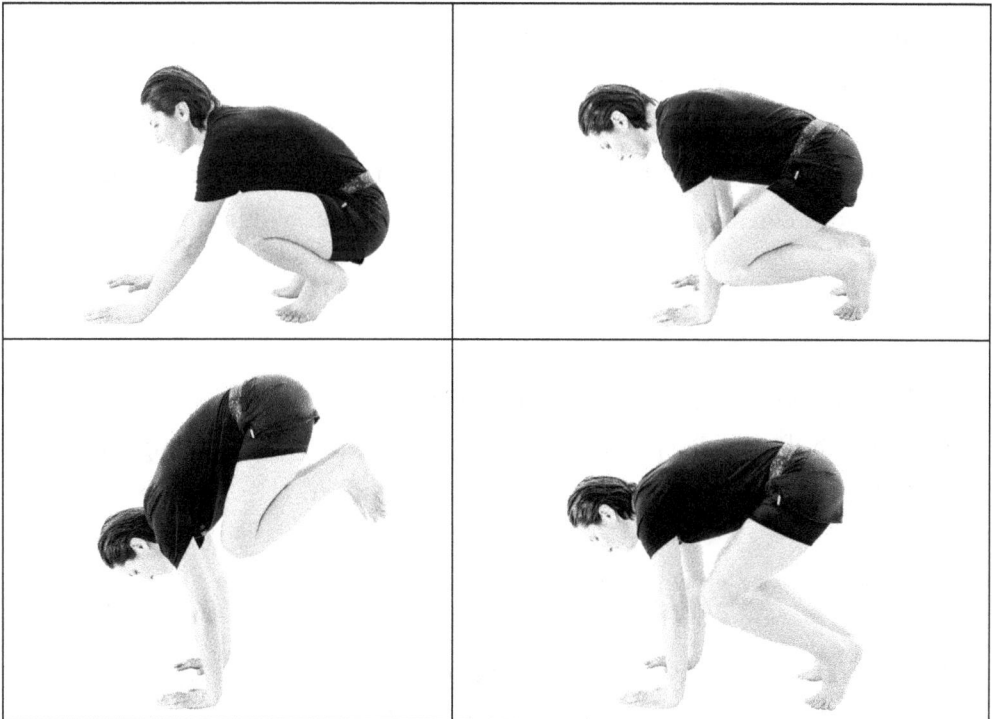

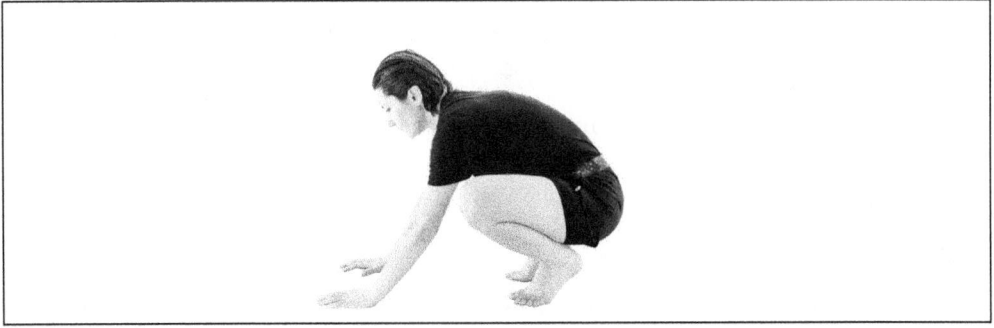

Frog Jump Spot

Aim to stay in the air for a fraction of a second and then use your abdominal muscles to place your feet back down.

The focus is not on how high you jump but on how soft and controlled your landing is and how long you can keep your body in the air. Landing should be graceful, without a sound, just like a Ninja or a feline. You will jump higher with time and practice. The focus is to learn to use your core muscles, to jump, leap, move and run "from your core".

If you struggle to lift your feet off the floor just transfer your bodyweight from your feet to your arms and back again. Keep trying to lift by tensing your core. With time your core and arms will get stronger and you will be able to take off.

Progression:

- hold the position in the air before coming down
- lengthen the landing phase – you can count, in seconds, how long it takes you to land and try to make that last longer and longer

Common errors and/or weaknesses to be aware of:

- Not transferring the body weight over the arms enough to "unlock" the legs . This can be due to a weak upper body. Work on just putting as much weight as possible on the arms without lifting the feet off the ground as mentioned before.

- Landing heavily. The upper body may not be able to support the weight yet or the core is not strong enough yet. Keep trying to control the movement as the muscles will grow stronger.
- Placing your hands too far forwards which causes an uncontrolled body weight transfer. Hands should be placed as far forwards as possible without the need to transfer the body weight until it is intended to do so.
- Placing only the top part of the hand on the floor, not the heel of your palm as well. The whole palm should be placed on the ground in front to support your whole bodyweight.
- Resting knees on elbows. Keep the knees away from the elbows and use your core instead.
- Knees are inside the arms. Knees should be outside the arms/elbows. They will be inside for another exercise, but for this one keep them out.

FROG JUMP FORWARDS

Benefits

The areas of the body involved are the same as those of the Frog Jump Spot and both frogs so far are working in the sagittal plane.

The only difference here is that you will workout your lower body more than in the first jump as you move forwards.

Technical points

You perform this frog jump in a similar way to the previous one. You lower yourself into a squat, rock onto your toes and keep your knees wide apart and your feet under your hips.

You then place your hands as far forwards as possible without shifting your body weight, and transfer your bodyweight onto your hands until your shoulders are over your wrists.

81

Lock in your abdominal muscles and gently and in a controlled way lift your feet off the ground without aggressively pushing off against the ground. Drive your feet forwards and squeeze the knees towards the chest.

Land slightly forwards from the original place, as close as possible to your hands, squeezing your tummy muscles.

As you lands place your feet softly back down, as opposed to dropping back on the ground without control.

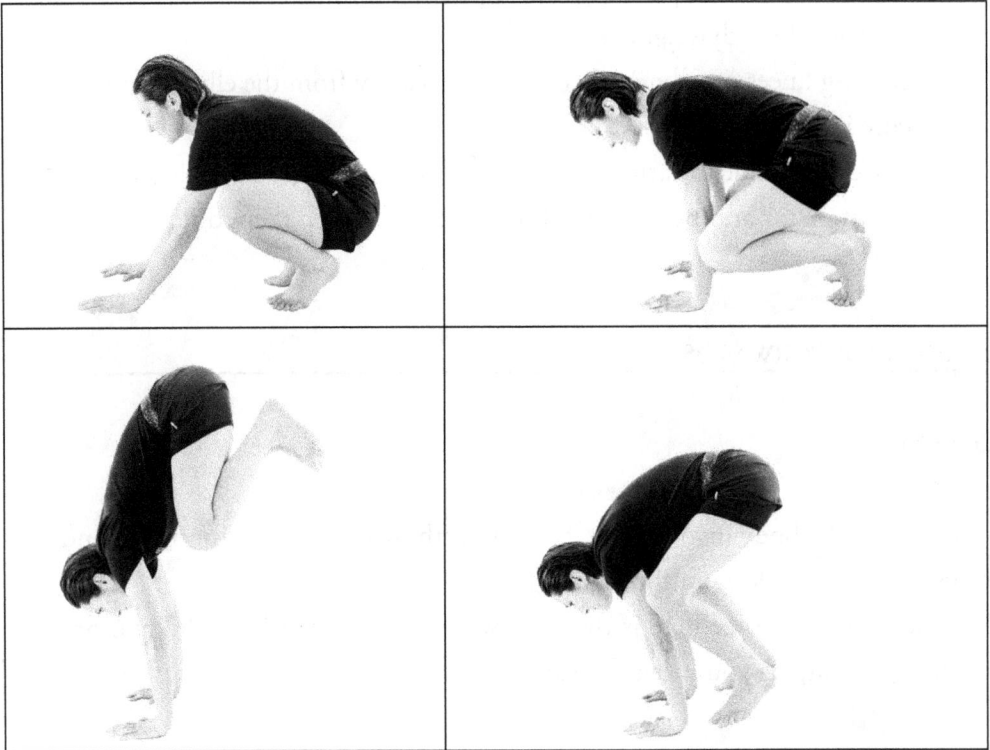

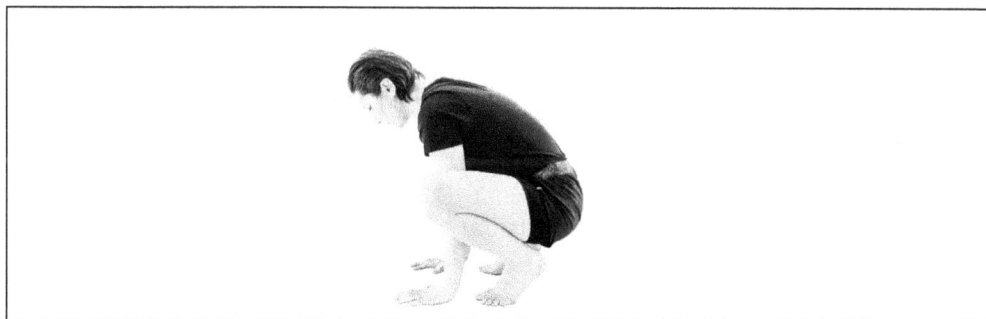

Frog Jump Forwards

As previously mentioned, aim to stay in the air for a fraction of a second and then use your abdominal muscles to gently place your feet back down. The focus is not on how high you jump but on how softly you land and with how much control.

Landing should be graceful, without a sound. Height comes with time and practice.

If you practise the spot one enough, the forward jump will come easier.

Progression:

- jump uphill
- jump faster and raise your heart rate as well; do this only after you understand the techniques or at the end of a session during the cardio phase which you will learn about later in the book
- jump backwards (see technique notes for Frog Jump Backwards)
- hold the position in the air before coming down
- lengthen the landing phase; you can count, in seconds, how long it takes you to land and try to make that last longer and longer

Common errors and/or weaknesses to be aware of:

The same points apply to this frog as for the Frog Jump Spot.

The only point to be aware of here is trying to jump too high or too far ahead (leaping) before understanding the technique. This causes uncontrolled landing and high impact; height and length are not important at the beginning. Understanding how to use the abdominal muscles to lift and place the feet back down is the first step, once this is understood and performed, speed, length and height can be addressed.

Furthermore, if you rush you won't get the strength benefits that come with slow, controlled movement. Not everything can or should be done fast.

Frog Jump Backwards:

Frog Jump Backwards requires even more control. Master the Frog Jump Forwards before going into reverse.

In reverse, ensure you don't jump too far back with your feet. You will know if you do because you will stretch so far you need to push off against the ground with your hands after landing.

When you figure out the correct distance to land with your feet, you will transfer your bodyweight onto your feet and gently lift the hands off the ground – there is no need to push off. It will become a smooth movement.

FROG JUMP SIDE

Benefits

The side frog jump works with the body's frontal plane.

This exercise benefits the body in a similar way to the previous frog jumps, the only difference is that the emphasis is on the strength of the obliques (the sides of the trunk), which are part of the core.

Technical points

The Frog Jump Side is the same as the forwards version, but you move to one side only, then switch to the other side.

As before, begin with the feet hip width apart, lower yourself into a full squat and rock onto your toes, keeping your knees outside your arms.

84

Here comes the difference. Place your hands on the ground a few inches to the side you want to move to, at a comfortable distance, where you don't need to transfer your body weight forwards or to the side until you are ready to perform the exercise. For the purposes of following instructions in a book, let's move towards the right side.

When you're ready to execute the exercise, shift your body weight onto your arms until your shoulders are aligned with your wrists. Nothing here is different from the other frog jumps. Lock in your abdominal muscles and gently and with control, lift your feet off the ground.

As you lift squeeze your knees towards your chest and land to the right side, behind your hands, not to the right of them, placing your feet softly back down.

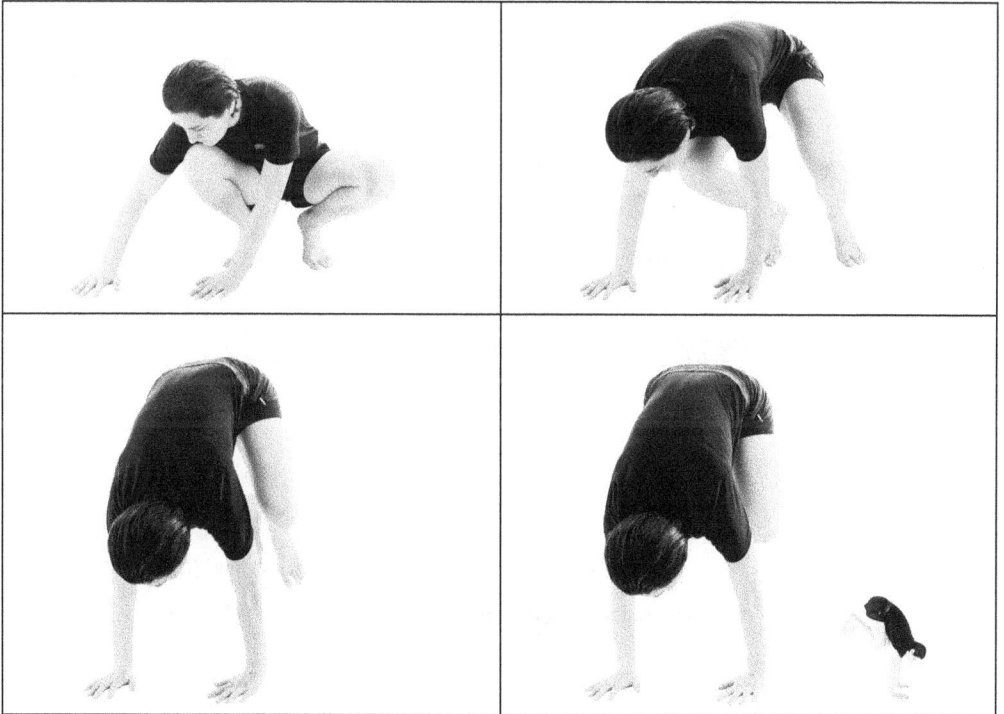

85

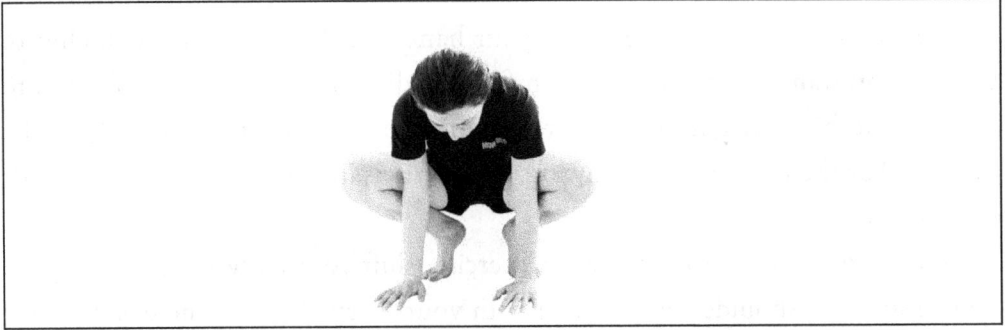

Frog Jump Side

Aim to stay in the air for a fraction of a second before landing. Landing should be graceful, with your focus on using your core muscles.

Repeat the same steps moving towards the left side.

Progression:

- hold the position in the air before coming down
- lengthen the landing phase: you can count, in seconds, how long it takes you to land and try to make that last longer and longer

Common errors and/or weaknesses to be aware of:

Take the points from the previous frog jumps and add a few more pertaining to this particular exercise.

- Placing hands too far to the side, which causes an uncontrolled body weight transfer. Hands should be placed just next to the foot. There is no need to overstretch.
- Placing the hands to the side and too far forwards ending up moving in a diagonal direction.

Landing ahead too far to the side of the arms. Aim to land right behind the hands and not to the side. This requires more control from the core than if you let your legs do whatever is comfortable for them.

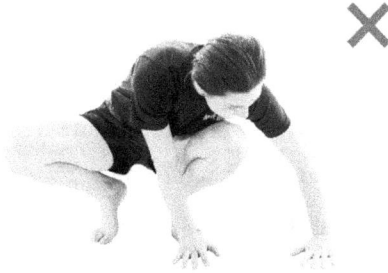

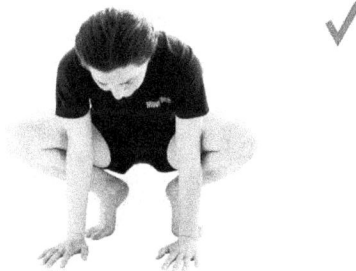

Frog Jump Side, landing

FROG JUMP TWISTED

Benefits

The added benefit of this type of frog jump is that works in the transverse plane of the body. That means it includes a rotation. This means increased core stability, strength, balance and coordination. There are many movements you do daily that include rotations, from picking your cup up with your right hand from your left side to picking up a box and turning around to look behind you, as well as working in the garden and playing with your children.

Furthermore, rotational movements improve mobility around your spine, which means reduced pain, and around multiple joints. With the twisted frog jump in particular, the rotation in your shoulder mobilises the joint in a way you wouldn't normally think of, and it's good to take the joint through various mobilisation movements.

87

Technical points

Begin with the feet hip width apart, lower yourself into a full squat and rock onto your toes. Keep your knees outside your arms at all times. Your toes can point outwards and heels inwards. Hold your feet under your hips with the knees pointing out. Nothing new for you so far, this is the start position for all the frog jumps.

Now, place the right hand on the ground, with fingers facing 180°, towards the way you will be landing after the twisted jump. Your hands should not be too far away from your body.

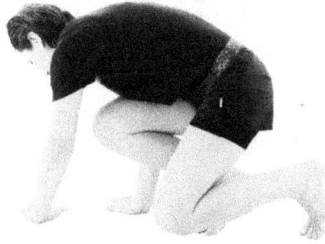

Frog Jump Twisted, twist starting position

Twist your body and shift your body weight towards the right, placing your left hand next to your right, about shoulder width apart. Allow the knees and feet to turn as they feel comfortable to allow for the body to perform the movement. You aim to turn or twist your whole body 180°, so upon landing you will be facing the opposite way, thus your hands must be positioned accordingly.

When you're ready to execute the exercise, shift your body weight onto your arms until your shoulders are aligned with your wrists, lock in your abdominal muscles and lift your feet off the ground in a controlled manner.

As you lift squeeze your knees towards your chest and land with your feet right behind your hands (not to the side) with knees outside your arms.

Frog Jump Twisted to right and left shows the whole movement from beginning to end, twisting to the right and then to the left.

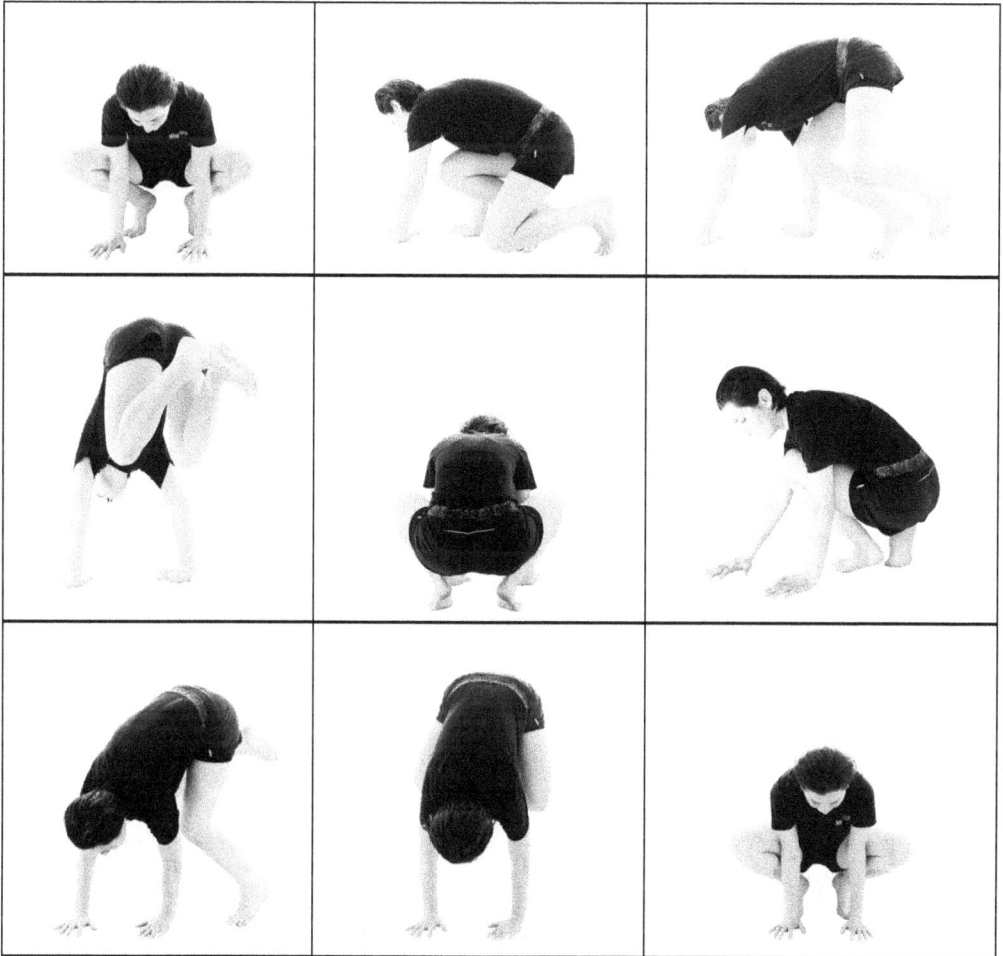

Frog Jump Twisted to right and left

Aim to stay in the air a little and your landing should be graceful as usual.

Continue twisting the left, right, left, right etc.

Begin with a few reps and perform them slowly. Build up to do more reps, still slowly, with a very good technique. Then move on to faster, higher and more reps, keeping the form for as long as possible. When you have lost form, stop, rest and resume. Keep this in mind for every single exercise in this book.

Progression:

- hold the position in the air before coming down
- lengthen the landing phase: you can count, in seconds, how long it takes you to land and try to make that last longer and longer

Common errors and/or weaknesses to be aware of:

- Hands are not fully facing 180°so the turn is not complete and you don't move in a straight line.
- Not rotating the body or transferring the body weight over the arms enough, which leads to pushing off and landing heavily.
- Landing heavily.
- Placing hands too far away from the body, which causes an uncontrolled body weight transfer. Hands should be placed near the body.

Also remember the points from the previous frog jumps.

TIGER WALK

Benefits

The Tiger Walk is an excellent upper body exercise. Similar to a press-up with integrated mobility and movement, this exercise strengthens your upper body including arms, shoulders, upper back and of course your core. What I find beneficial here is the fact that the core engages in different positions and areas thus creating that all-round core strength.

Apart from the obvious strength benefits, this exercise also lightly stretches the hip flexors and improves hip mobility. You will see as you transition or walk forwards or backwards that your hip is involved in the process.

Technical points

Begin with a squat, as always. With your feet hip width apart, lower yourself into a full squat, rock onto your toes and then into a press-up position, with your wrists under your shoulders.

Activate your core, pull your belly button in, place the right hand forward, further than you would in a Panther Walk and the opposite foot, your left foot, forward but to the side of the body. Your left knee faces out to the side, not forwards or down towards the ground underneath you. Your left foot is resting on the inside of the big toe (allow the outside of the foot to lift off the ground).

Make sure your left leg is not underneath your body and the knee is not pointing up (it points forwards). This keeps the space under your body so that you can lower yourself into a press-up. In other words, ensure the inside of the left thigh is almost parallel to the ground.

Your left hand is under your body, with the shoulder over the wrist. Your right hand is in front of you.

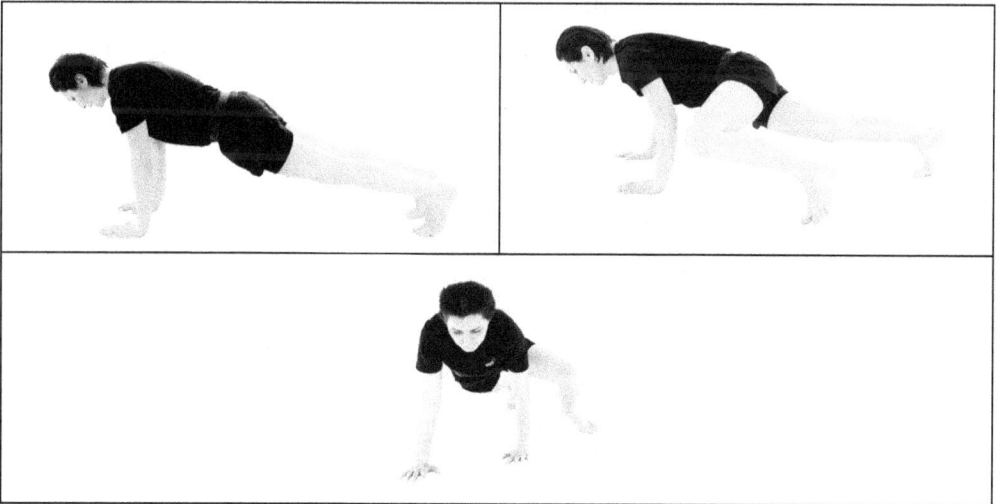

Tiger Walk, starting position side and front

To summarise the main points of the starting position and the position you will find yourself in throughout the exercise:

1. Back leg is straight, front leg bent.
2. Front foot is to the side of the body, with the inner thigh parallel to the ground and the outside of the foot off the ground. Knee points forwards.
3. The hand opposite the front leg is in front of you. The other hand is under the body and the shoulder is aligned with the wrist.
4. Your bodyweight is evenly distributed between your arms and legs.
5. The bent leg has a rough angle of 90°at the hip and at the knee. Too high and your knee reaches your face, too far back and you won't be able to smoothly transition to the next position.

It's important to get the basic stance right as this is where most people get tangled up. So take your time and feel the position you are in right now. When you are ready continue with the press-up.

Leading with your chest, bend your elbows and perform a press-up. Look in front of your hands when you perform the press-up, do not allow your head to hang down. Hips stay in line with your chest. When you do a press-up in general, remember this: chest leads, hips follow.

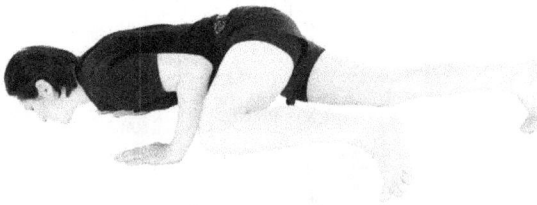

Tiger Walk: press-up

Looking at *Tiger Walk press-up* observe how the bent leg (left) has the thigh parallel to the ground to allow for the hips to move down. If the thigh is not parallel to the ground it will look like *Tiger Walk, front foot.* That is anything but a press-up.

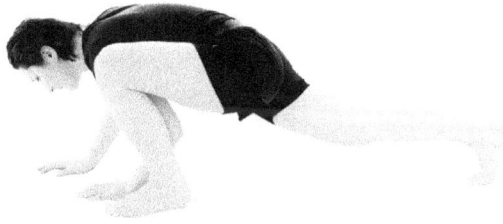

Tiger Walk, front foot

It's the same for the front foot. If it is fully placed on the ground and not on the inside of the big toe, your press-up will look like *Tiger Walk, front foot*. If the foot is fully on the ground, the knee can only go upwards and we go back to the point I made above about the knee.

Similarly if the forward knee is under the body and not to the side, your press-up will not have room and it will look like *Tiger Walk, knee under body*.

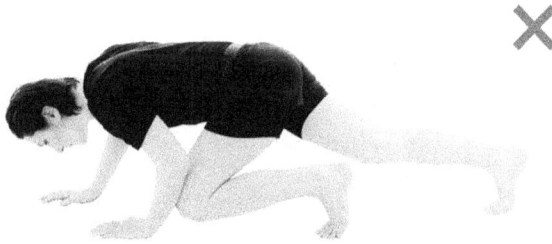

Tiger Walk, knee under body

In *Tiger Walk, press up*, observe the front leg and the rough90°angles at the thigh and knee compared with *Tiger Walk, front foot* and *Tiger Walk, knee under body* where there are no right angles.

Moving in the Tiger Walk

You should have the left foot and right hand forward. Check your position to ensure you can follow the instructions from here on.

Step forward with your right leg, twice as long as a panther stride, and your left hand stretches in front of your body.

When stepping forwards your legs will travel twice as long as your hands so avoid moving the arm first. Instead straighten your front leg and launch yourself forwards with your back arm, stretching as far as you can.

Tiger Walk movement shows the full transition from right hand forwards to left hand forwards. Observe the distance travelled, the position of the back hand and that of the front hand. Observe in the top right-hand picture how the left arm stretches almost at the same time the left leg straightens.

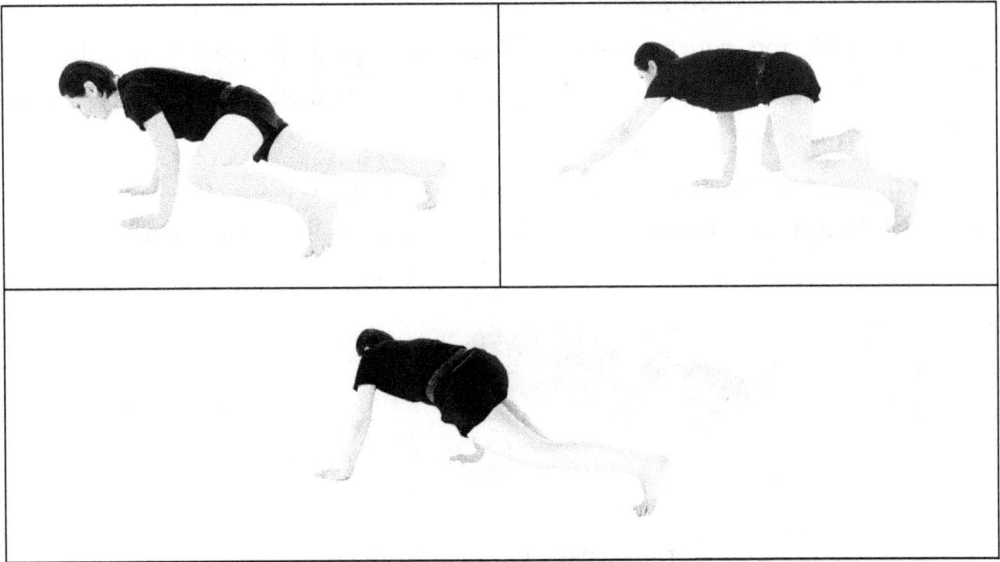

Tiger Walk movement

If you position your hand first and then step with your foot, your position will look like *Tiger Walk, hand first*. There is no room for the back leg to straighten and the front leg to step forwards. As the legs naturally travel further than the arms, the arms need to stretch out quite a bit to make room.

After each step you will, of course, perform a press-up, then move forwards to another press-up.

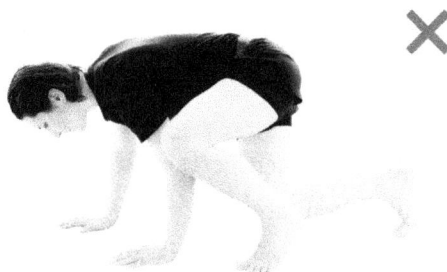

Tiger Walk, hand first

Breathing

It is important to be aware of your breath and to use your breath to your advantage. Breathing correctly helps your body to activate the muscles needed to perform an effective press-up and feeds the muscles with oxygen.

When performing a press-up the general rule is:

Breathe OUT on the effort, when you PUSH UP.

Breath IN when you lower yourself DOWN.

Breathing out deflates the stomach and contracts the abdominal muscles. Use your abdomen to push you up, as a platform would.

- *Push UP – Breathe OUT*
- *Go DOWN– Breath IN*

Common mistakes and/or weaknesses to be aware of:

- Back leg is bent. Your back leg should be almost straight.
- Front leg is under the body or the knee points up instead of to the side. This places the leg in the way of the chest, the hip cannot move down so the press-up cannot be performed (*Tiger Walk, front foot* and *Tiger Walk, knee under body*).
- When stepping forwards, the front hand is not far enough to allow room for the back leg to make the long stride. This leads to either lifting the hips up in the air, bending the back leg or moving the back leg backwards to straighten it (*Tiger Walk, hand first*).

95

- Hips are too high when performing the press-up. Hips should follow the chest which leads the movement; don't leave them behind or lower them ahead of the chest.
- Sinking into the shoulders when performing the press-up. Shoulders should be activated to stabilise them and lock them in place.
- Head is hanging down or lifting to look ahead. Keep in mind that the neck should be straight and the eyes should point just in front of the hands.

Notes:

It does not matter how low or high you perform the press-up at the beginning. Focus on technique, depth will come with practice as you grow stronger. That doesn't mean you shouldn't push yourself, you have to push yourself to get stronger. What I'm saying is build the correct technique, then push yourself while keeping the technique.

Focus on the chest leading the way down and allow the hips to follow. When the chest stops, the hips stop as well. Imagine there is a platform underneath you which moves up and down with you and lifts you up as one unit or as a straight plank.

Tiger Walk can also be performed backwards. In the Move Wild video library, you can see the movement performed backwards.

THE CROCODILE

The Crocodile is a multilateral training exercise based on press-up variations. Instead of doing the same press-up over and over again, you vary the position every time.

The general rule is: with the legs completely straight, perform a press-up every time you move one hand.

Benefits

As expected from a press-up-based movement, the Crocodile strengthens the upper body (i.e. arms, shoulders, upper back and core).

On a secondary level it improves wrist and ankle mobility and strength.

Most importantly the multilateral way of performing the press-ups allows your body to learn how to adapt to different positions. You build all-round strength and your body will be able to react faster to sudden changes in movement and maintain its strength. This is useful for example when you lose your balance.

By training in a multilateral way, you develop reflexes to efficiently and effectively react to various situations.

Technical points

Begin, as you are used to, with feet hip width apart. Lower yourself into a full squat, rock onto your toes and into a press-up position. Your wrists are positioned under your shoulders and your abdominal muscles are activated. Perform a press-up where you are right now.

Next, move one hand somewhere else on the floor, in a different position, while keeping your legs straight. The feet can move around to adjust for the press-up position but the legs are always straight. You are essentially walking in a plank position in between press-ups. The forwards, backwards and side movement comes from the ankles and not from bending your knees. Perform another press-up in the new position.

Move the other hand around, anywhere, maybe with fingers facing a different way. Move your legs and feet accordingly, keeping legs straight. Press-up.

Move the other hand, in a different position. Adjust your feet. Press-up.

Continue moving your hands all over the place and each time one hand moves, perform a press-up. Don't move both hands at once.

You're aiming for as many variations as possible. Try to see how many unique positions you can place your hands in.

In *The Crocodile, hand positions,* you have a few examples of hand positions. Every time one hand moves it is followed by a press-up. Also notice how the torso and hips turn as well.

Avoid moving hands only forward and back, try to get creative and move them around, everywhere, in as many positions and facing as many directions as possible.

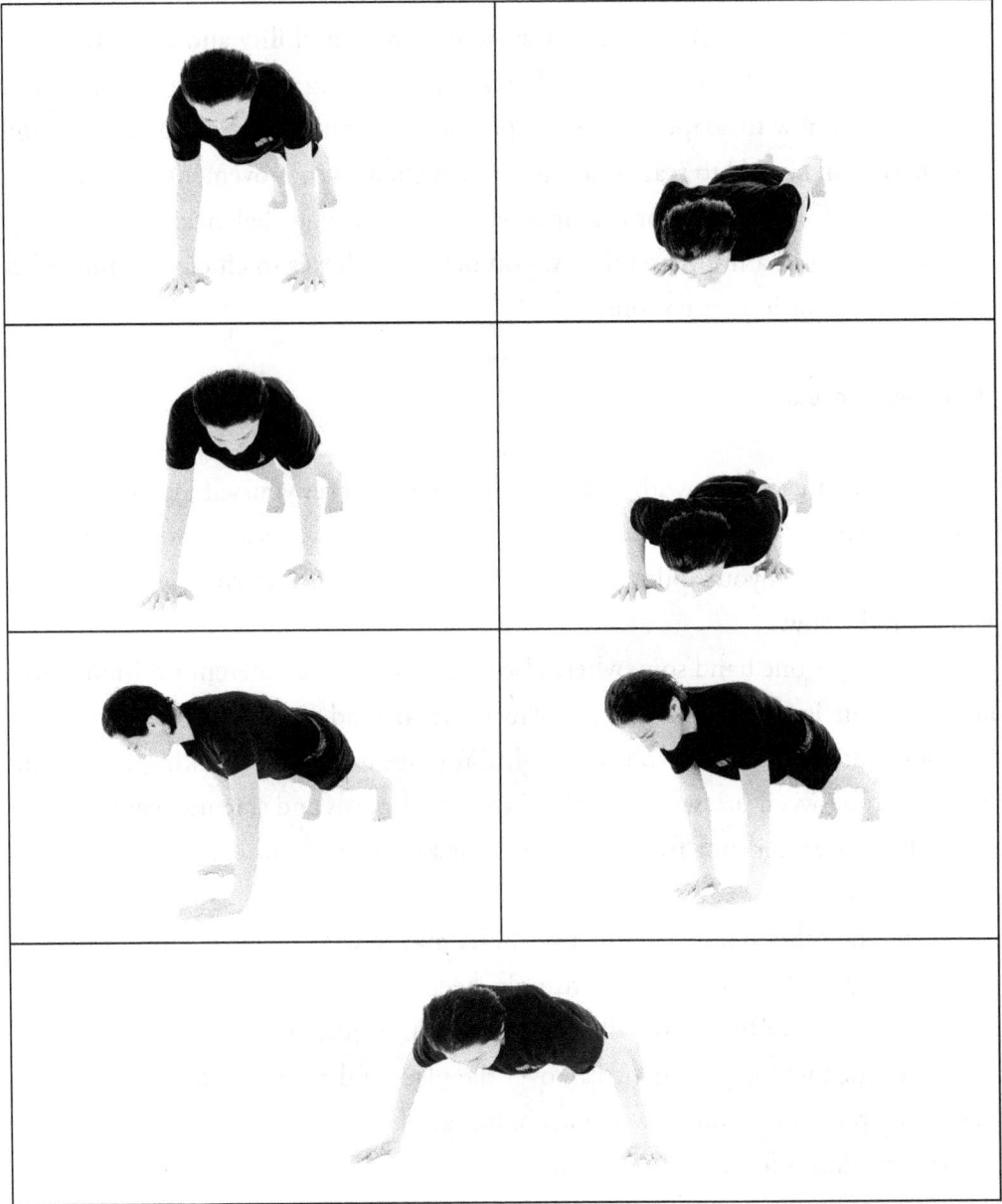

The Crocodile, hand positions

Common errors and/or weaknesses to be aware of:

- Knees are bent (*The Crocodile, errors* top left). Keep your knees straight and move around like you would in a plank.
- Hips lift too high (*The Crocodile, errors* top right) or drop too low (bottom left). The chest guides the movement: the hips should follow the chest. Whatever height the chest stops at, that's where the hips stop as well.
- Head hanging down (*The Crocodile, errors* bottom right) so the neck is not straight. Look just in front of your hands, not down, not forwards.

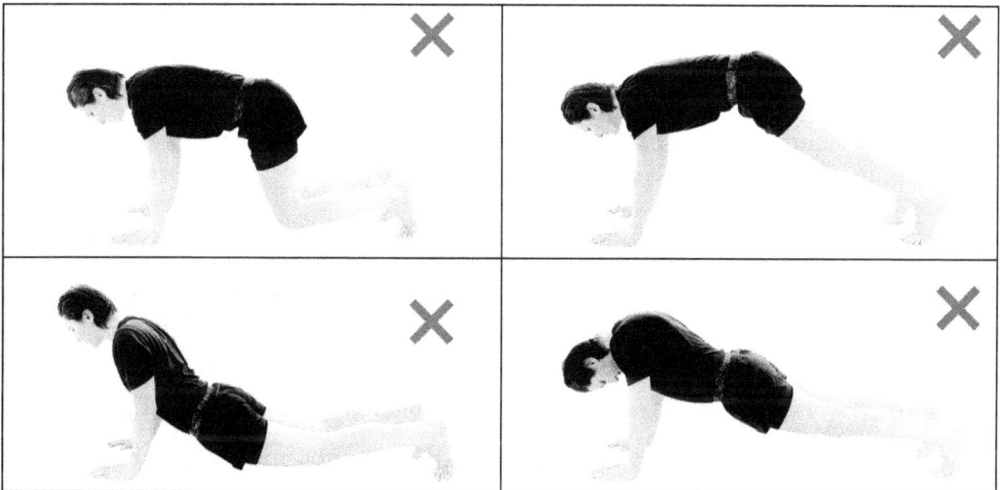

The Crocodile, errors

Notes:

It does not matter how low you go into the press-up. It can be an inch, but make that inch correct. Once it's correct, you can push yourself harder.

As a general rule you want your elbows to brush the sides of your body when they bend. In the Crocodile exercise you are working with variations on a press-up and this will not always be possible. However it's good to remember that when performing a classic press-up with the hands placed shoulder width apart, your elbows should brush the sides of your body.

Get creative, move your hands:

- Forwards and backwards
- In and out to the side
- Place your hand underneath your body and form a triangle shape with your thumbs and index fingers
- Turn your wrists and fingers to point in different directions
- Place your hands far away from your body, under your body or shoulder width apart
- Combination of the above
- Move hands clockwise and anticlockwise

DUCK WALK

We may remember this movement from when we were children. It may have had a different name but it's the same. The only difference between then and now is that now you are using this exercise in a more mindful manner, for the benefits it brings when performed in a controlled fashion.

Benefits

The Duck Walk strengthens the quadriceps, core, foot and ankle muscles, knee and hip stability muscles.

It improves balance and mobilises the ankles, feet and hip while taking the joints through their full range of motion.

What I love most about this exercise is the ankle mobility and core strength. If you do it right, and don't let your foot go out to the side, you will feel your core working hard. So let's see how we can achieve this.

Technical points

Begin with the feet hip width apart, lower yourself into a full squat, rock onto your toes and place the right foot in front with the heel on the ground, as if talking a step.

Your left heel is lifted off the ground, abdominal muscles are activated and your back is leaning very slightly but it's straight, not hunching over.

When stepping forwards, gradually transfer your body weight onto the right foot. You cannot move the back leg until you shift 100% of your weight onto the front foot.

As you transfer the body weight onto the right foot, drop the left knee down very close the ground (without touching the ground) and then squeeze it up to your chest straight away. The left foot moves straight forwards and under your body, not out to the side, if possible.

You will feel tension in your abdominal muscles when you squeeze the knee to your chest, like an ab crunch, if you keep your body straight and move the back foot under your body and not to the side. If you slouch there is no room for the knee to lift and the foot will go out to the side, so keep your body straight.

Duck Walk shows the whole process, moving from right foot forwards to left foot forwards. To get the most out of this exercise, do your best to keep your body straight and move the back foot under the body, like the wheels of a car, and not out to the side.

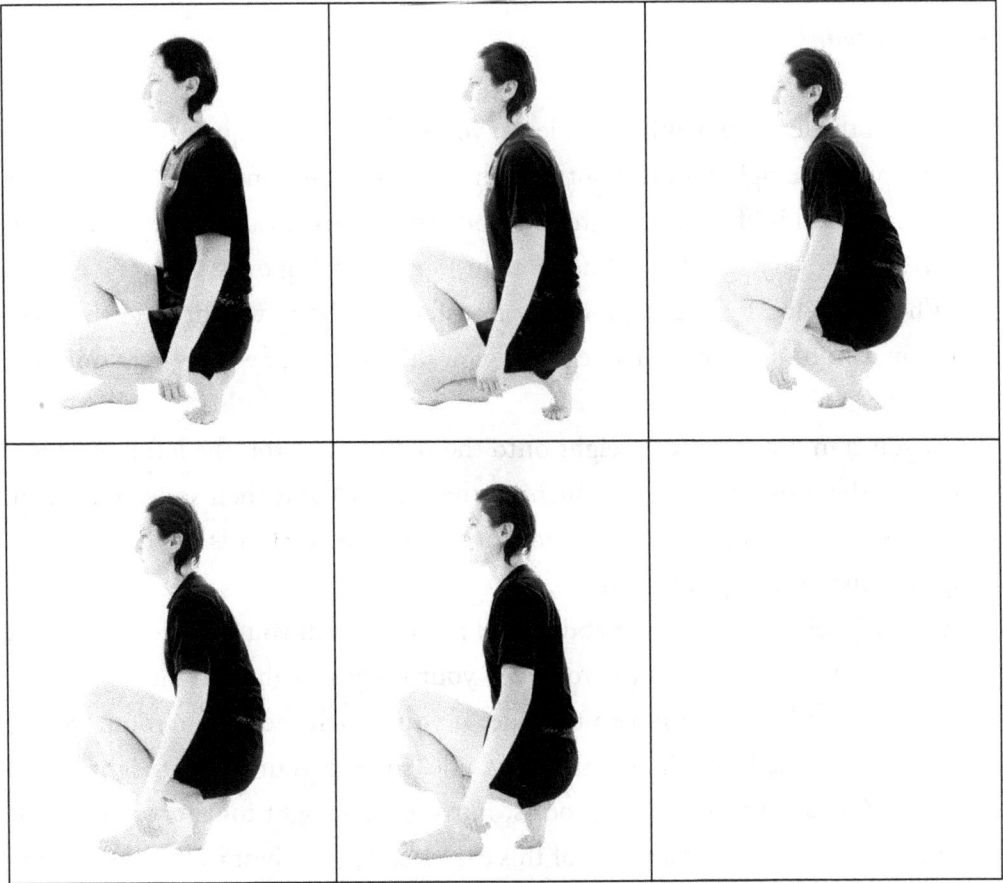

Duck Walk

Step with the left foot forwards, place the whole tripod on the ground and continue walking, this time dropping the right knee very close to the ground, then squeezing it up to the chest and stepping with the right foot forwards.

Continue transferring the body weight and walking. The slower the better for your balance and mobility training.

Duck Walk Backwards

Walking backwards is the same but you need to fully transfer your bodyweight onto the back foot until your front foot can easily come off the ground. When there is almost no weight on it, you can lift it off the ground.

Common errors and/or weaknesses to be aware of:

- Feet move out to the side instead of forwards and under the body. This is common at the beginning, but as you progress, your feet should move forwards, not to the side as in *Duck Walk, foot out to the side.*

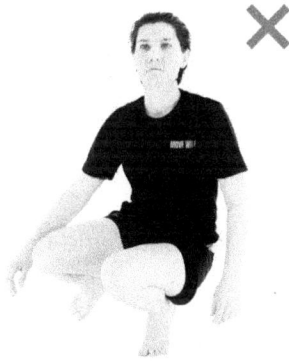

Duck Walk, foot out to the side

- Slouching. There should be a slight lean at the hip but the back should be straight, just not necessarily vertical. If you slouch there is no room for the knee to lift to the chest.

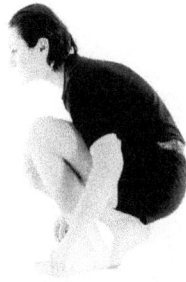

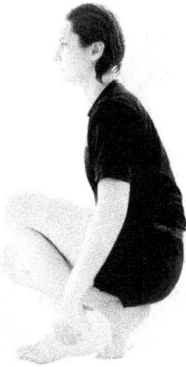

Duck Walk, slouched and not slouched

- Placing hands on the ground to recover or maintain balance. Again this is common at the beginning, and it's not necessarily wrong, just inefficient. As stability muscles and balance improve, your hands should not make contact with the ground anymore.
- Front heel comes off the ground. Ensure you ground the front tripod before moving on. It can lift once you step forwards.

SPLIT SQUAT

Benefits

The Split Squat strengthens the major lower body stability muscles. These include the quadriceps, glutes, adductors, abductors and core.

It also strengthens the smaller joint stability muscles in the feet, toes, ankles, knees, hips. By now you know that these stability muscles require a different approach to strengthen them rather than aggressive and fast exercises.

This movement also mobilises the ankles, knees and hips, taking the joints through their full range of motion.

Technical points

With feet hip width apart and toes facing forwards take a step forwards with the left foot, about half of your normal stride length.

With your body lengthened, abdominal muscles activated, looking forwards and with a straight back and a neutral spine, ground the left foot and slowly bend the knee, going down into a Split Squat. Allow the back heel to lift off the ground.

If you can't keep your front heel on the ground the stride is too short, so move the foot forwards slightly. As the front foot is fully on the ground, most of your weight is on the front, so when you stand up (next step), ensure that you place most of the weight and pressure on the front foot.

Time to perform the actual squat, but before you stand up be mindful of the following aspects:

1. **Root the front tripod** into the ground and push up through your heel (keeping the toes on the ground). As you stand up, if you keep your back straight you will feel your glutes activating.
2. **Squeeze the thighs together** to recruit the adductors and stabilise your stance. You don't actually need to touch the thighs against each other, it is possible to tense the adductors without bringing the legs together.
3. **Activate your core.** This will enable you to hold your posture.

4. **Clench your buttocks** as you come up – imagine you have a platform under your backside lifting you up. Remember the difference between clenching and tucking.

After activating and recruiting the correct muscles you can perform the squat and stand up. You should be in the same position you started with.

Then take a step forwards and follow the same pattern: tripod, squeeze thighs, core, clench, stand up.

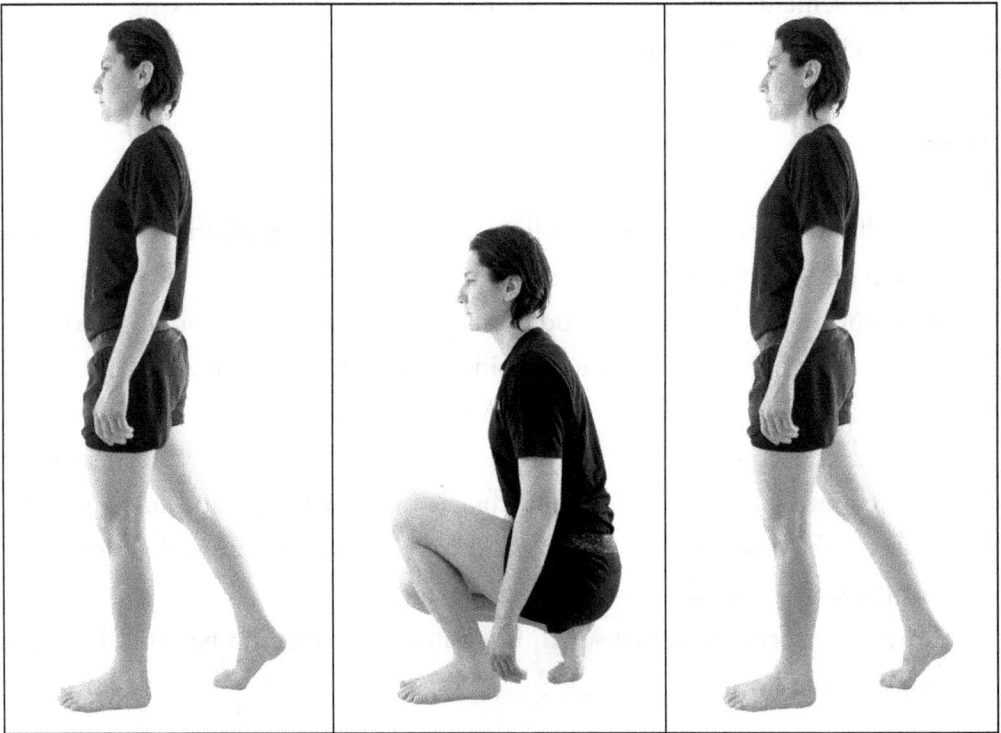

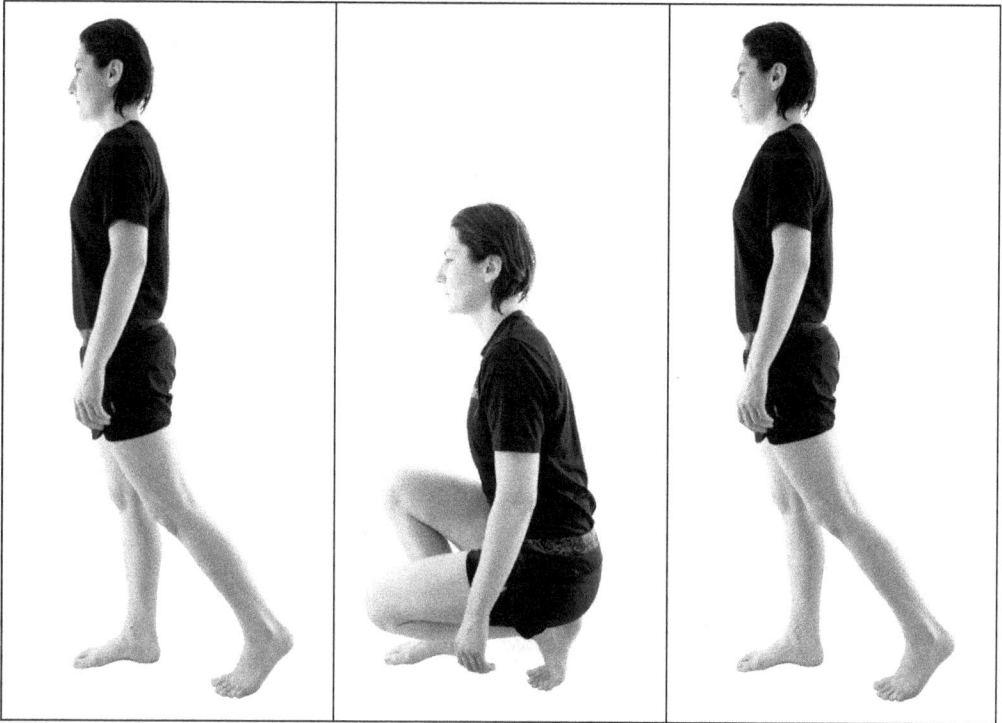

Split Squat

Throughout the movement ensure that:

- Your trunk is as straight as possible. If you find this difficult and you need to lean forwards, it might be that your glutes or core aren't strong enough yet. If you struggle you can always come back to this movement once you get stronger through practising the others. Return to this exercise from time to time to see the progress.
- Your abdominal muscles are tensed throughout.
- You breathe out on the effort (i.e. when you stand up), and breath in when you lower yourself down.
- The front knee tracks the front foot, doesn't collapse inward and doesn't push out.
- The movement is smooth and continuous without any jerks or different speeds.

This is of course ideal. However, don't worry if you can't be mindful of all these points at the same time. Take each point and focus on it for a few reps, then take another point and focus on that. In time your body and nervous system with begin to remember and will be able to do all of these things at the same time. Enjoy!

You can also perform the Split Squat backwards. The same technical points apply.

Common errors and/or weaknesses to be aware of:

- Front knee buckling or pushes out to the side too much. This places strain on the knee joint and surrounding tissues. The front knee should track the foot. See *Split Squat, knee buckling.*

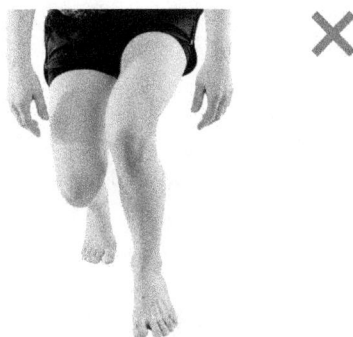

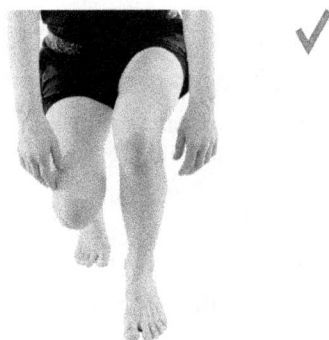

Split Squat, knee buckling

- Front heel lifts up. This means the front foot is too close to the body and the ankle may not yet be flexible enough. Move the foot slightly forwards and ground the tripod.
- Leaning forwards excessively as in *Split Squat, leaning forwards*. This is common for beginners in particular as they don't have the strength and cannot recruit the correct muscles; it can also happen with trained individuals who may not know how to recruit the correct muscles, are rushing or are tired but they keep going. When technique breaks down too much it is better to stop before bad habits creep in.

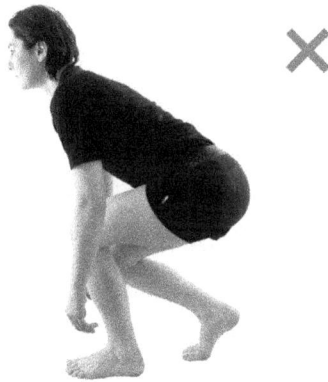

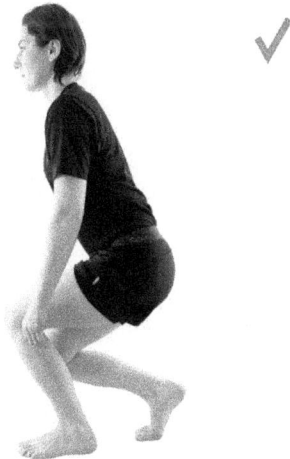

Split Squat, leaning forwards

- Jerky movements. This may indicate muscle weakness at some point in the movement; you usually feel this at the bottom of the squat when there is a sudden drop and/or on the way up from the bottom to about half-way.
- Too much weight is being placed on the back foot and leg. The back foot is mainly for support, it takes less of the weight because it's not firm on the ground. The front foot, however, is rooted into the ground, so it is this one that should support the bulk of the weight.

Notes:

Breathing is very important in this exercise, as it is in all movements. It is worth repeating the pattern here.

The breathing pattern for the Split Squat is similar to that for a press-up. **Breathing out is on the effort**. When the out breath is done correctly the abdominal muscles activate; in fact all the core muscles activate.

The general rule is to **breathe out on the effort**. Always remember this because it can helps in your day to day movement. When the abdominal muscles need to tense, breathing out will achieve this.

CROSS FROG

Benefits

As an advanced version of the Frog Jump, the Cross Frog is extremely good for all-round core strength.

It also strengthens the upper and lower body and the stability muscles in your feet, ankles, knees and hips for better balance, stability, control and general movement.

This exercise also mobilises the wrists, hips, back, knees and ankles and improves coordination and agility.

Technical points

Begin in a standing position, squat down with the heels on the ground, then rock onto your toes.

Place both hands in front of the body, as you would in a Frog Jump stance and thread the right leg through the gap between the left hand and left foot. Place the left heel (underneath you) on the ground. You can lift the left hand off the floor if you wish.

Cross Frog, starting position shows you the starting position (top photo) and the position with the right leg threaded, from the side and front (bottom photos).

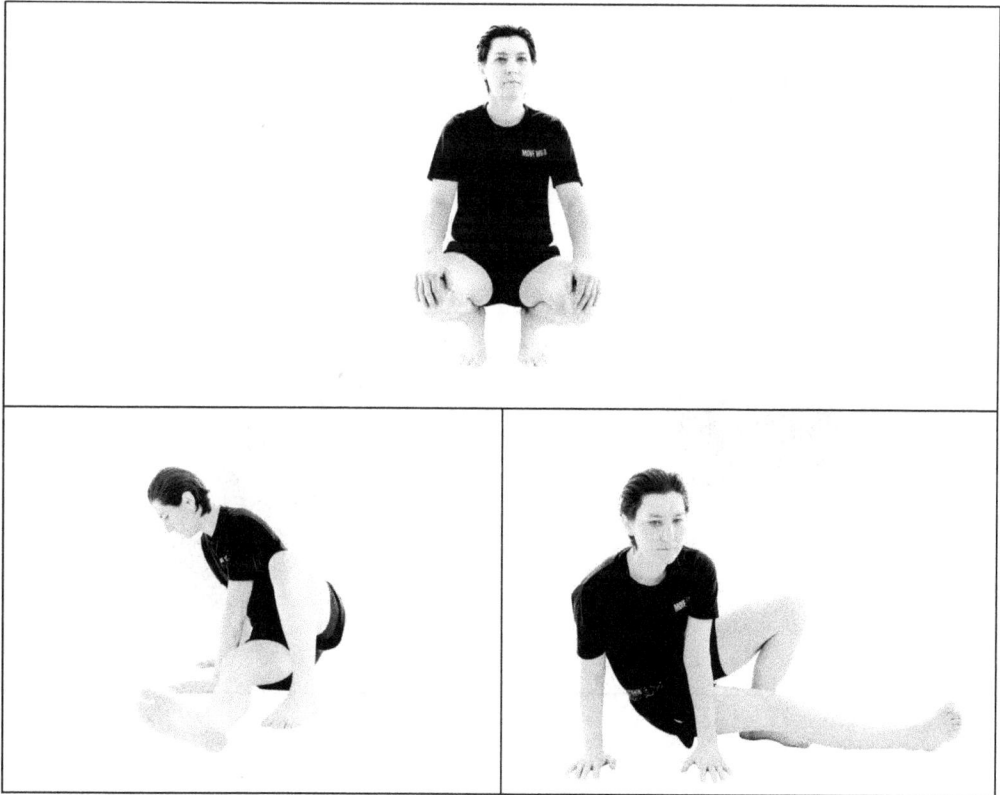

Cross Frog, starting position

From here, pull the right leg under your body (the same way it went out), place the left hand further forwards than the right (so you're moving forwards), and thread the left leg through the gap between the right leg and the right hand.

You should now have your right leg under you (heel on the ground) and your left leg stretched out.

Cross Frog step by step shows you the step by step movement. The top 4 images show you the movement from the side. The 4 bottom images show you the same movement from the front.

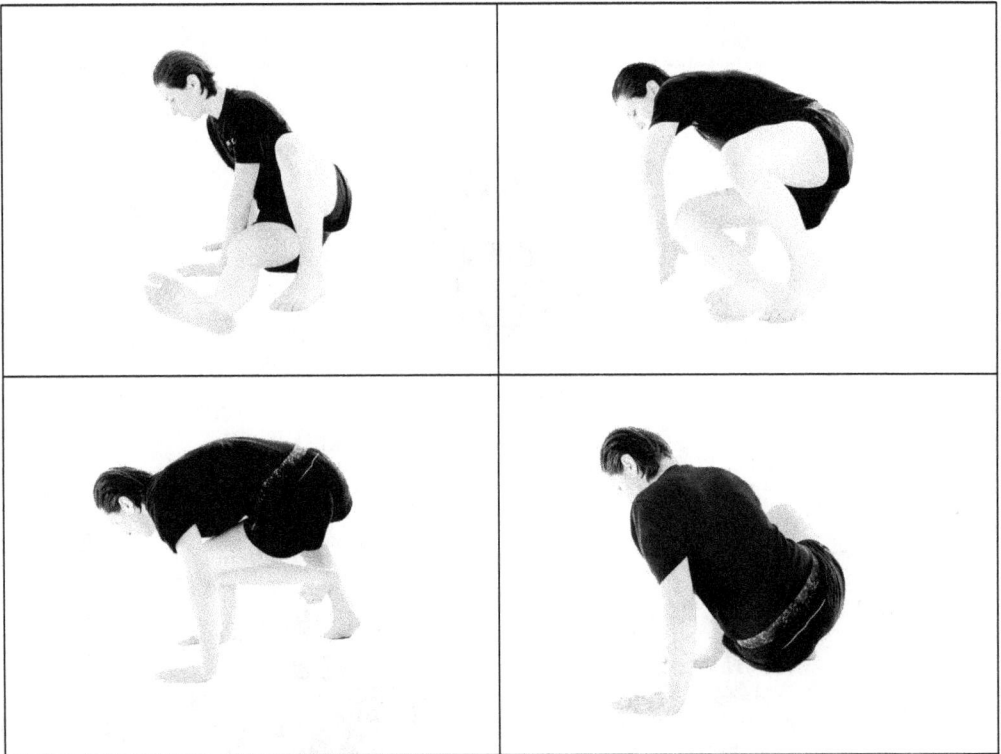

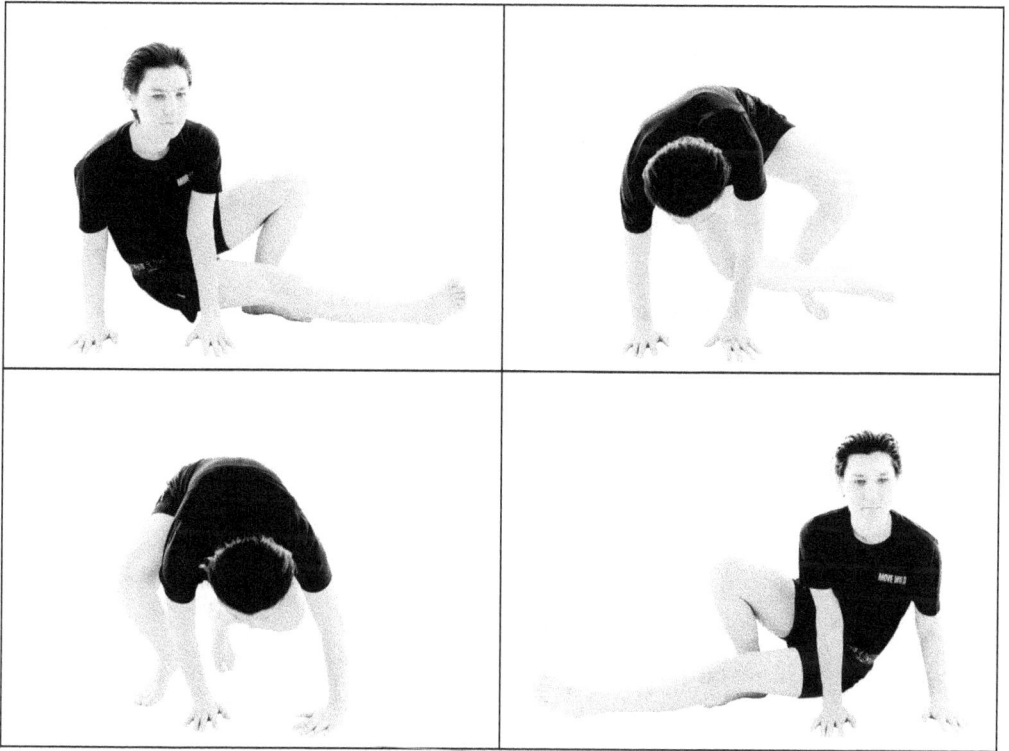

Cross Frog, step by step

Now repeat on the other side. Pull the left leg under your body, place the right hand in front of the left, twist and thread the right leg through. You should have your left leg under the body and your right leg stretched out, as in the start position.

Keep changing from side to side and building momentum. Then try to switch sides by jumping. To make it easier try to:

- Perform the movement without a jump, just place the feet on the ground one by one
- Perform the movement with a jump but on the spot
- Perform the movement without a jump, on the spot

Progression

- Perform the movement jumping backwards. Same technical points apply but the hands move all the way back, almost under the body.
- Increase speed and/or number or reps

Common errors and/or weaknesses to be aware of:

- Foot closest to the body is up on the toes and/or too far away from the body. Heel should be on the ground and close to the body, almost under the hip.
- Not transferring the body weight over the arms enough to unlock the legs. This can be due to poor upper body strength.
- Placing hands too far away from the body. When you perform the jump you have little support if you stretch out too much.
- Trying to jump too high before understanding the technique. This can lead to a heavy, uncontrolled landing and high impact. As with almost every other exercise in this book the focus is on building technique first. In this case height is less important at the beginning. Once you understand the movement, you can jump higher, faster and further.

MONKEY SHUFFLE

Benefits

Another excellent exercise for core strength. We are in the more advanced movement section of this book so everything is a little bit more challenging, of course depending on your level of fitness. The Monkey Shuffle looks like the Panther Walk sideways. It strengthens the core, the obliques in particular, as well as the upper and lower body as a whole. It's exceptional at improving coordination and agility and, performed at speed, it trains the cardiopulmonary system as well. Again an all-round exercise which I personally like very much.

Technical points

From a standing position, squat and rock onto your toes, as for all of these exercises.

Place yourself in a press-up position with wrists under your shoulders, then walk your feet forwards until the knees are under your hips. Activate your core muscles. You should be in the familiar Panther Walk position.

While holding the knees bent, an inch above the ground, hips low and wrists under the shoulders, move to your right by crossing the left hand over the right and move the right out. Then shuffle – left foot in, right foot out (close/open).

Monkey Shuffle, step by step shows the movement from the front and side. Look closely at how the hands and feet move. Try to follow.

This sequence can be altered after you learn the movement and can do it fast and correct. Make it yours. For now follow the pattern to learn it and build your agility and coordination.

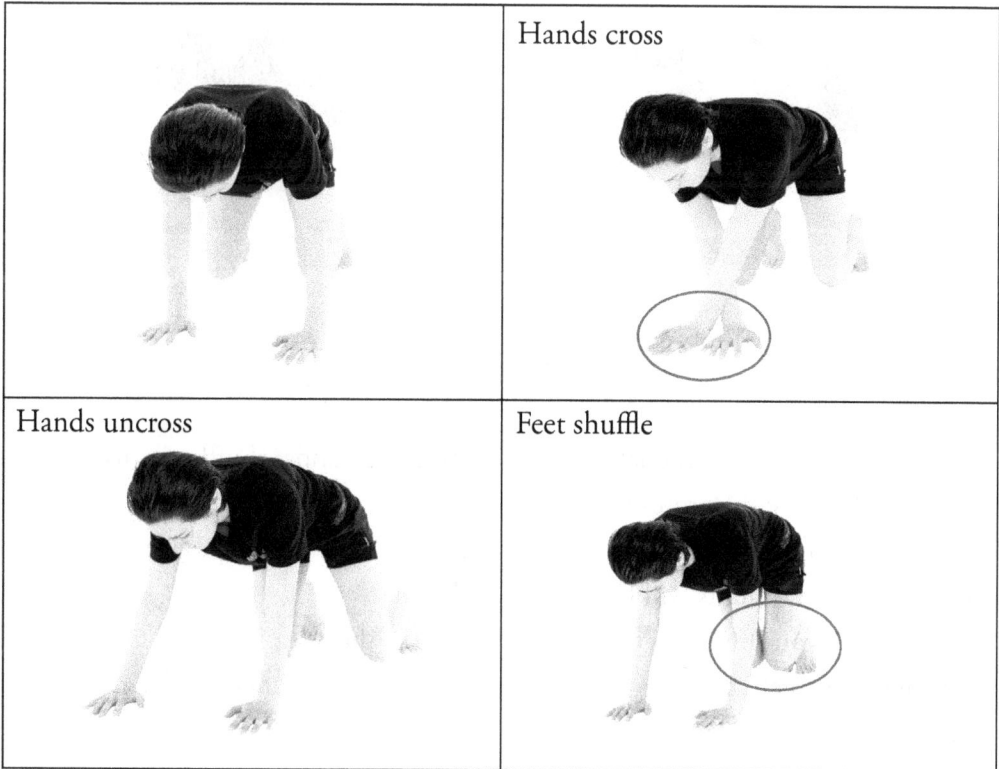

	Hands cross
Hands uncross	Feet shuffle

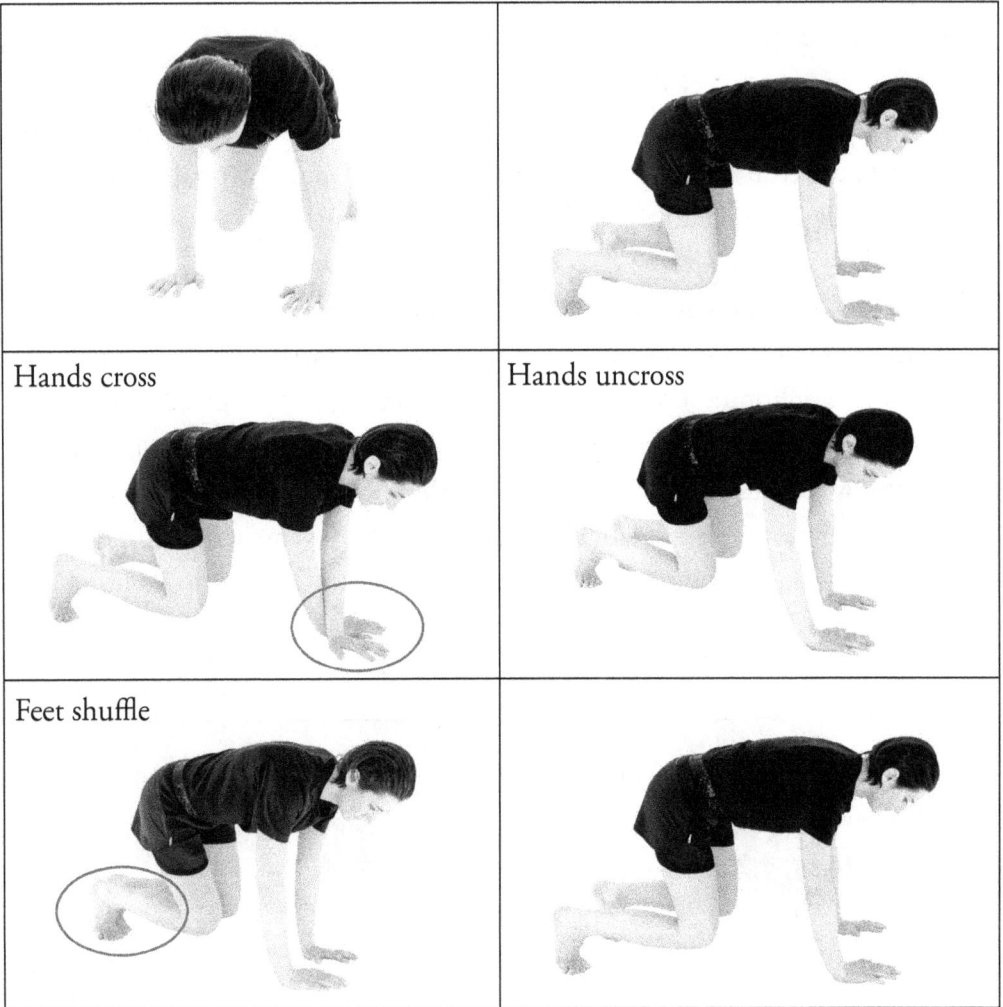

Hands cross

Hands uncross

Feet shuffle

Monkey Shuffle, step by step

Continue with the same sequence cross/uncross the hands, shuffle the feet. Don't jump, shuffle above the ground.

As you get better and faster you don't need to keep this sequence, it will just flow and the movements will blend into each other.

Make sure you shuffle to the right and then to the left.

When you feel confident with the movement sequence perform it faster and faster while holding the form described above. See how long you can keep your form:

- knees under the hip and an inch above the ground
- hips low
- wrists under the shoulders
- looking right in front of your hands; keeping your neck straight
- cross the hands, shuffle the feet
- The aim is to move fast, smoothly, lightly and fluidly while keeping your form as best you can.

Common errors and/or weaknesses to be aware of:

- Jumping instead of shuffling. This may happen when you begin to speed up; remember to keep your knees about an inch off ground. This should prevent you from hopping.
- Stretching arms too far in front and/or legs too far behind. Keep wrists under the shoulders and knees under the hips. This will help you not to stretch the stance too much and to stay compact.
- Lifting knees and hips too high. This allows your body to relax the core somewhat which you don't want. You want the body to use the core and to move from the core, so ensure your knees are just an inch above the ground and your hips are not high in the air.

Bunny Hop

The Bunny Hop is similar to the Frog Jump but the knees are inside the arms and tight together, as opposed to outside the arms.

Benefits

The Bunny Hop tones and strengthens the upper and lower body, with emphasis on the shoulders and especially the core.

It also strengthens the stability muscles and mobilises the wrists, hips, back, knees and ankles as do many of the exercises in this book.

Technical points

As always, begin with feet hip width apart, lower yourself into a full squat, rock onto your toes and place your hands on the ground in front of you at a comfortable distance so that you don't need to transfer your body weight forwards at all.

Your knees are inside your arms and squeezed together, with the toes and knees pointing forwards.

When you're ready to execute the exercise, shift your body weight onto your arms until your shoulders are over your wrists. Lock-in your abdominal muscles and gently, with control, lift your feet off the ground, as opposed to pushing against the ground or jumping. Squeeze your knees under your chest.

Land slightly forwards from the original place and as close as possible to your hands. As you land, place your feet softly back down, as opposed to dropping back onto the ground without control.

Hold your knees together throughout the exercise as much as possible, it forces the core to activate.

Bunny Hop, step by step shows the exact sequence, including the bodyweight transfer in the 2nd picture of each row, from the side and front. Observe how, once the hands are on the floor, the knees are together and they stay this way throughout the movement.

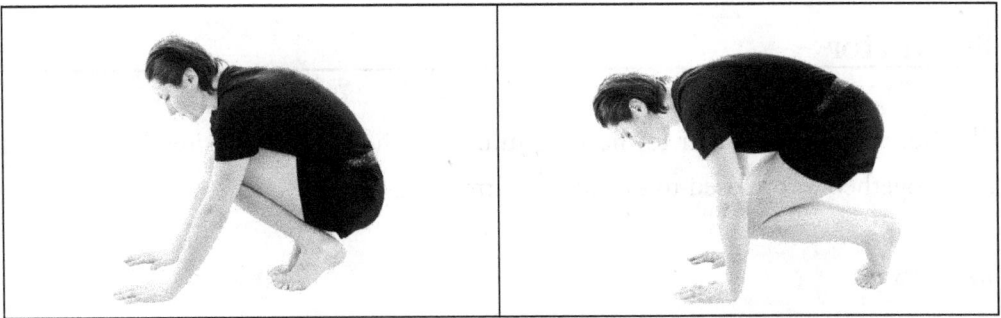

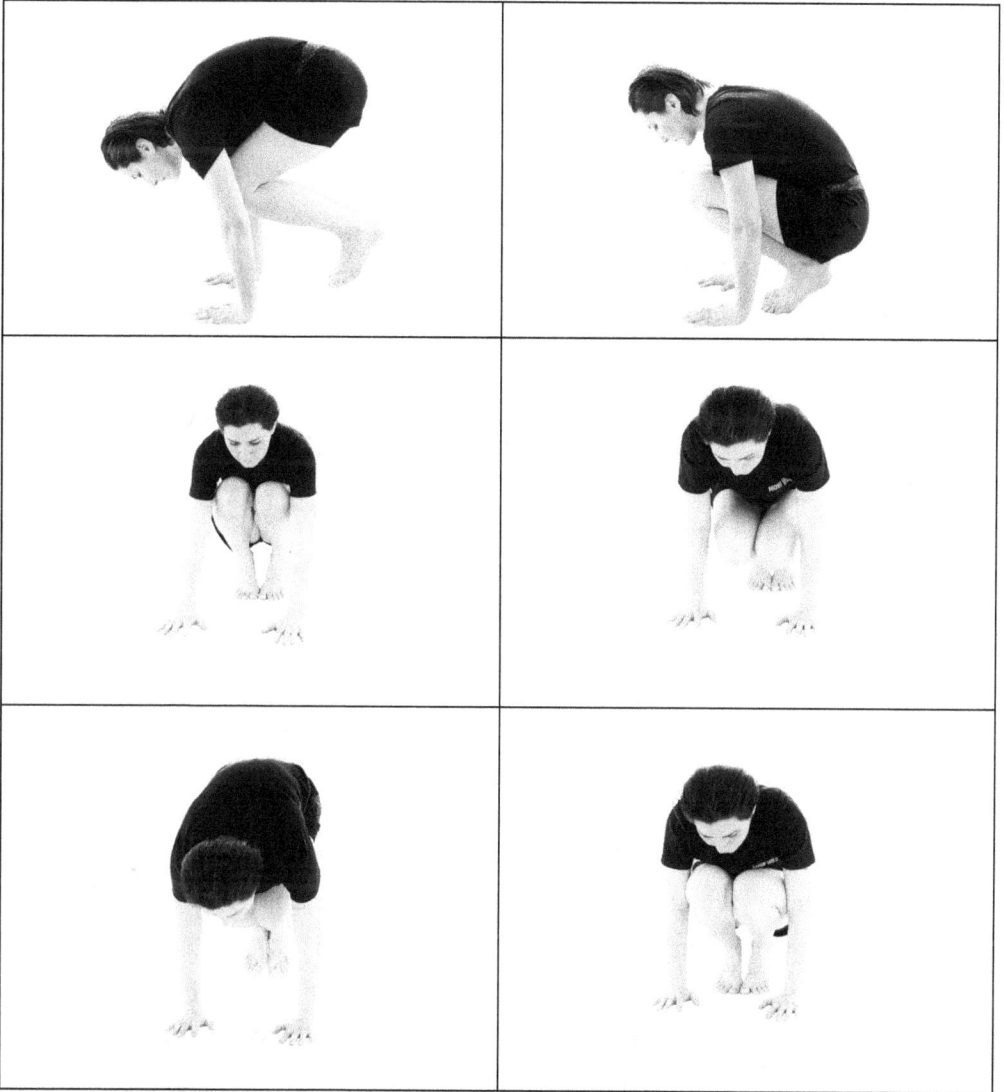

Bunny Hop, step by step

Aim to stay in the air for a fraction of a second and then use your core to place your feet back down. Focus not on how high you jump but on landing softly, with control, and on keeping the knees together throughout the movement.

Landing should be graceful. You will jump higher with time and practice. The focus is to learn how to use your core muscles; to jump, leap, move and run from your core.

Common errors and/or weaknesses to be aware of:

- Knees outside the arms.
- Knees not held together throughout the hop, like in *Bunny Hop, knees apart*. The closer your knees are from start to finish, the more effective the exercise is. However, don't worry if you can't do this from the start. You will not injure yourself if you keep your knees apart.

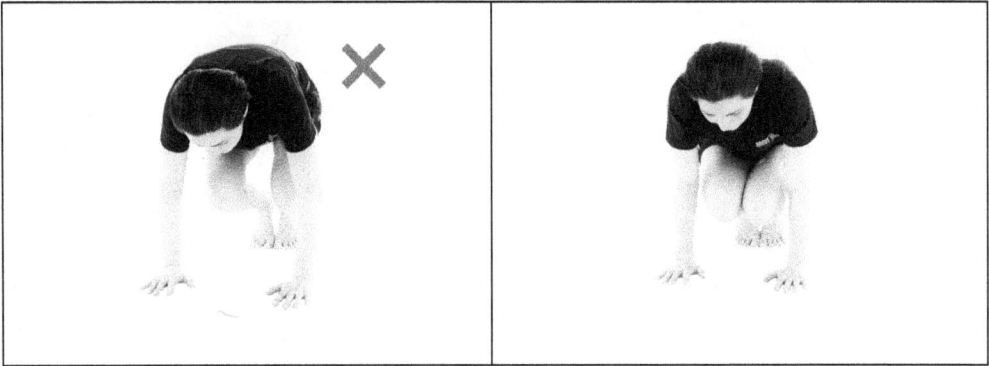

Bunny Hop, knees apart

- Not transferring the body weight over the arms enough to unlock the legs. This makes it difficult to lift the feet off the floor. Ensure your shoulders are above the wrists before you "hop".
- Landing heavily. This could be because the upper body may not be able to support the weight yet or the core is not strong enough yet so the control is not there. In this case, either go back to the previous exercises and return to this one from time to time, or keep practising a few reps every time you perform your Move Wild routine. Either option works and in time, with practice and perseverance, you will get stronger, more flexible and more agile.
- Placing hands too far forwards, which causes an uncontrolled body weight transfer. Hands should be placed as far forwards as possible but without the need to transfer the body weight until you intend to do so.

Notes:

The Bunny Hop is particularly good for abdominal muscle strength. Try to squeeze the knees as far forwards as possible, aiming to get the feet in between the arms and crunching the abdominal muscles.

To make that happen, place a sheet of paper between the knees and try to keep it from falling. This will help you keep your knees together throughout the movement. You will notice the difference.

BALANCE AND BODYWEIGHT TRANSFER

Balance exercises can be dangerous if you lose your balance. Make sure you do not practise them in a crowded or cluttered room. Ensure that if you lose balance you do not fall onto something that might lead to an injury. Do not assume that you will not lose balance. Choose an open space with plenty of room and free of hazards. Remember, safety first.

With balance and bodyweight transfer exercises, the slower you move the better. These are excellent exercises to help strengthen stability muscles throughout the body. Thus we are aiming for focused and mindful movement.

Move Wild comprises 7 fundamental balance and bodyweight transfer exercises. From these, variations can be created or other forms of exercise brought in. The fundamental Move Wild balance and bodyweight transfer exercises are:

1. Standing Body Weight Transfer
2. The Clock
3. 360 Degrees
4. Seesaw
5. Prone Body Weight Transfer
6. Supine Body Weight Transfer
7. Prone to Supine Flow

Let us take each exercise and understand what is does and how to do it to get the most out of it.

Remember you have all these exercises at www.movewildacademy.com/move-wild (password "duckwalk").

STANDING BODY WEIGHT TRANSFER

This exercise aims to bring awareness of side to side body weight distribution and to teach how to use stabiliser muscles.

There are 3 stages to this exercise. The first is performed from a natural standing position, with feet hip width apart and toes pointing forwards, transferring the body weight from one leg to the other while standing with correct alignment and knees slightly bent/soft.

The second is transferring the body weight from one leg to the other while holding a squat position with thighs parallel to the ground or as close to that as possible.

The third is performed from a crouched position or a low squat for those who are able.

Keep in mind that not everyone has the necessary control to go to the 3rd stage, or even the 2nd. This is absolutely fine. Keep working on stability muscles using other exercises and come back to these to see how the level of control has improved.

Benefits

This simple exercise, going through all the stages, can strengthen your ankle, knee and hip stability muscles, as well as the major stabilisers such as the quadriceps and glutes, adductors and abductors.

It strengthens the core, particularly when you reach the more difficult stages and, of course, improves balance.

Technical points

Stage 1

Standing with knees slightly bent/soft, root the tripods (heel, little toe, big toe) into the ground and elongate the body from the crown of your head. Whenever either foot or both feet are on the ground try to be mindful of this stance.

Keeping your back straight, abdominal muscles tensed, glutes clenched and always looking forwards, slowly and gradually shift your body weight to one foot, without lifting the other foot off the ground.

As you transition ensure that your knees do not collapse inwards and aim for slow, fluid, uninterrupted movements. There should be no pushing or jerky movements.

It helps to think about the percentage of weight being transferred from one foot to the other. For example if you transfer to the right foot you can either count up from 0% to 100% of body weight being distributed on the right foot or you can think about the weight coming off the left foot and count from 100% to 0%.

Breathe normally throughout and feel the weight pushing against the floor as you gradually put more and more weight on one side of the body.

Keep transferring your bodyweight from one foot to the other for a few minutes and then move onto Stage 2.

Stage 2

From a standing position, tripod on the ground, back straight, with correct alignment and lengthened body, lower yourself into a squat until the thighs are almost parallel to the ground. Hold this position throughout the exercise, unless you take a break, in which case stand up as you would from a squat (i.e. with the back straight and bodyweight evenly distributed on both feet).

To avoid pushing off or any jerky movements you will use your trunk and arms as counterbalance to gradually transfer the bodyweight from one foot to the other.

To transfer the bodyweight onto the left foot you need to lift your left foot off the ground first, so you can step to the left. But to lift it you need to take the

123

weight off. To do this transfer all your body weight onto the right foot and lean your trunk and stretch your arms to the right to counter balance. Stretch as far as you need to, until the weight comes off your left foot.

Try to keep your trunk straight even when bending from the hips, and look forwards. You will feel your abdominal muscles working very hard, tense them and contract your buttocks(particularly the right) to stabilise the position (do not tuck, clench instead). By activating the glutes you also ensure that the hips don't go out of alignment.

When you feel that the left foot is almost coming off the floor, lift it, stretch it out further to your left and slowly and gradually begin to shift your weight onto it.

Similarly, in order to bring your right leg in, next to the left, you have to transfer all your body weight onto the left leg to unlock the right foot so you can lift and move it. To do this, transfer the body weight onto your left foot and reach with your trunk and arms to your left as far as you can, to counterbalance.

When you feel the right foot almost coming off the ground, pick it up and bring it closer to the left. You should still be in a squat position.

At this point you can:

1. Stand up and reset, then go back into the position and move to the left again or to the right.
2. Continue shuffling to the left.
3. Move back to the right following the same instructions in the opposite direction.

As you transition, ensure that your knees do not collapse inwards (especially the knee you place all the weight on). Keep your abdominal muscles and glutes tensed, and aim for slow, fluid, uninterrupted movement. There should be no pushing off or jerky movements.

It helps to think about the percentage of weight being transferred on one foot or from one foot to the other as you did in Stage 1.

Breathe normally throughout and remember to breathe out on the effort.

Stage 3

From a standing position, with the tripod on the ground, correct alignment and lengthened body, lower yourself into a full squat. If it's difficult to hold your heels on the ground, rock onto your toes and perform the exercise in this crouched position. However, ideally you should be in a full squat.

To avoid pushing off or jerky movements you will use your trunk and arms to counterbalance, similar to Stage 2. Now the counterbalance is even more important as the stance is less stable, especially if you have your heels off the floor.

To move to the left, transfer all your body weight onto the right foot and lean your trunk and stretch your arms to the right to counterbalance. Stretch as far as you need to until you take all the weight off the left foot. At this point you will need to engage your core muscles to stabilise and maintain the position.

When you feel the left foot is almost coming off the floor, lift it and place it out to the left and slowly and gradually begin to shift your weight onto it.

To bring your right leg in, next to the left, you have to transfer all your body weight on the left leg. As you shift the body weight onto the left leg, reach with your trunk and arms to your left as far as you can, to counterbalance. When you feel the right foot coming off the ground you can pick it up and move it closer to the left.

At this point you can:

1. Place your heels on the ground, stand up through a squat and rest or reset, then go back into the position and move in whatever direction you want.
2. Continue stepping to the left.
3. Move back to the right following the same instructions in the opposite direction; so you take a step to the left, then right, then left and so on. This is particularly useful if you find yourself in a small space.

Ensure that your knees are stable and do not collapse inwards, keep your abdominal muscles and glutes tensed, and aim for slow, fluid, uninterrupted movement. There should be no pushing off or jerky movements.

It helps to think about the percentage of weight being transferred onto one foot or from one foot to the other as with all the balance transfer exercises so far. Breathe normally throughout.

Common errors and/or weaknesses to be aware of:

- Knees are shaky and/or collapse inwards. This is probably due to weak stability muscles which strengthen by doing balance exercises as well as exercises such as squats and lunges performed in a correct manner.
- The hip goes out of alignment on the support leg. Again, this may be a sign of weak stability muscles, especially glutes. Activate the corresponding side of the glutes and root the tripods into the ground.
- Pushing off. If you can't bring the foot in without pushing off, just transfer as much body weight as possible without letting the knee collapse, hold for a few seconds, and then transfer it back, without actually moving the feet. Sometimes the problem is that you don't actually transfer your whole body weight and thus cannot smoothly shift from one foot to the other. To help you with this, imagine you are reaching for someone's hand in front of you.
- Slouching. There is a bend from the hip as the arms reach out to counterbalance, but the back in not rounded. This is more challenging in Stage 3, however in Stages 1 and 2 the back should not be curved at all.
- Holding the breath. Breathing out on the effort, when transferring the bodyweight, helps to tense the abdominal muscles and help with stability and balance.
- Looking down. The eyes are a guide for the head and the head is a guide for the body. Where the eyes go, the head and body follow. Ensure that you look ahead and not downwards.
- Lifting shoulders too high towards the ears/hunching the shoulders. Shoulders should stay relaxed. There is no need for extra tension.

THE CLOCK

The Clock is a balance exercise where you imagine you are the centre of a clock and, balancing on one leg, you slowly move the other leg around the clock, tapping at each number all the way around. All your body weight is on the balancing leg, the centre of the clock. There should be no weight on the tapping leg.

Benefits

The Clock is excellent for strengthening your foot, ankle, knee and hip stability muscles. These are essential when trying to correct certain imbalances, as when performing slow movements, all weaknesses and imbalances come to light. When performed correctly this exercise can address and correct some of these imbalances, if not all.

It also strengthens the quads, adductors, abductors and gluteus muscles, which it turn stabilise the hip and knee.

It obviously improves balance, as well as posture, postural awareness and focus. This can help in situations when you would use your balance. You will be more likely to be able to swiftly recover your balance or even control your fall. Good balance is essential to movement.

To maintain balance you should focus on also using your core muscles. Thus the core is working as well.

This exercise can reduce the risk of injuries such as ankle sprains or knee pain by strengthening stability muscles and mobilising the joints.

It can potentially speed up recovery from injury by strengthening the stability muscles and correcting subtle imbalances as well as mobilising the joint.

Technical points

As usual, begin by aligning the body. Feet are hip width apart, the outside of the feet pointing forwards, toes slightly inwards, knees soft, tail bone slightly tucked in, ears aligned with the shoulders which are aligned with the hips which are aligned with the ankles. Elongate the spine and relax your shoulders, arms and hands.

Distribute your bodyweight evenly on both feet and between the front (ball of foot and toes) and back (heel) of each foot.

Imagine you are the centre of a clock. Gradually transfer your bodyweight onto the right foot. Bend your right leg slightly and ensure the tripod is rooted into the ground. Activate your abdominal muscles and tense the right buttock so the right side of the hip doesn't push out to the side, out of alignment, and both hips are level. Keep elongating the body and looking forwards while the nose, solar plexus and belly button are connected by a straight line, stacked on top of each other (i.e. do not lean back, forwards or to the side).

We will call this the Crane position; you can see it in *The Clock, start,* 1st and 3rd pictures from the left.

Imagining you are the centre of the clock, gently stretch your left leg out and tap the ground with your toes at 12 o'clock, in front of you. Do so without placing any weight at all on your left foot, you just tap the ground and slowly pull the foot back; 100% of the weight is on your right foot all the time.

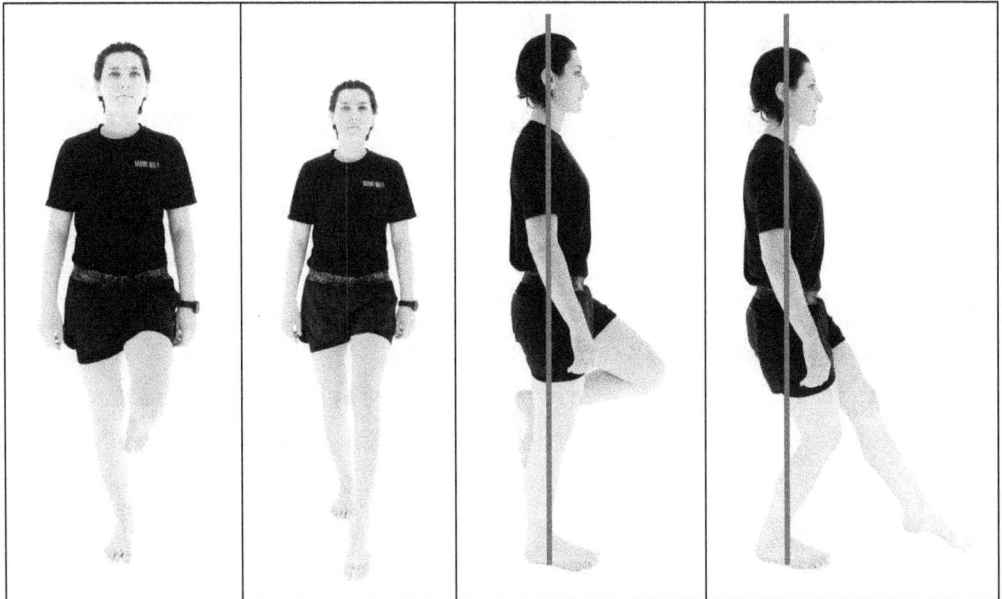

The Clock, start

Reach as far as you can without changing your alignment, your tripod, bodyweight distribution or losing balance. If you go too far and lose balance or make any changes to your posture, try tapping a little closer to your centre for the time being.

The only part of your body that should move is the left leg. You can also bend your support leg slightly when you reach out. However pay special care not to transfer your bodyweight off the tripod and onto the balls of your feet or toes. Ensure that you keep your heel rooted into the ground.

The movement is slow, controlled and fluid. The slower you move the better. If you balance on the right leg, continue by tapping, counter clockwise at 11 o'clock, 10, 9, 8, 7, 6, 5, 4, 3 (behind your right leg). For 2, 1 and back to 12, tap in front of the support leg. After each tap go back to the Crane then reach out for the next number.

The Clock, all the way round shows parts of the Clock when balancing on the right leg for a few of the numbers.

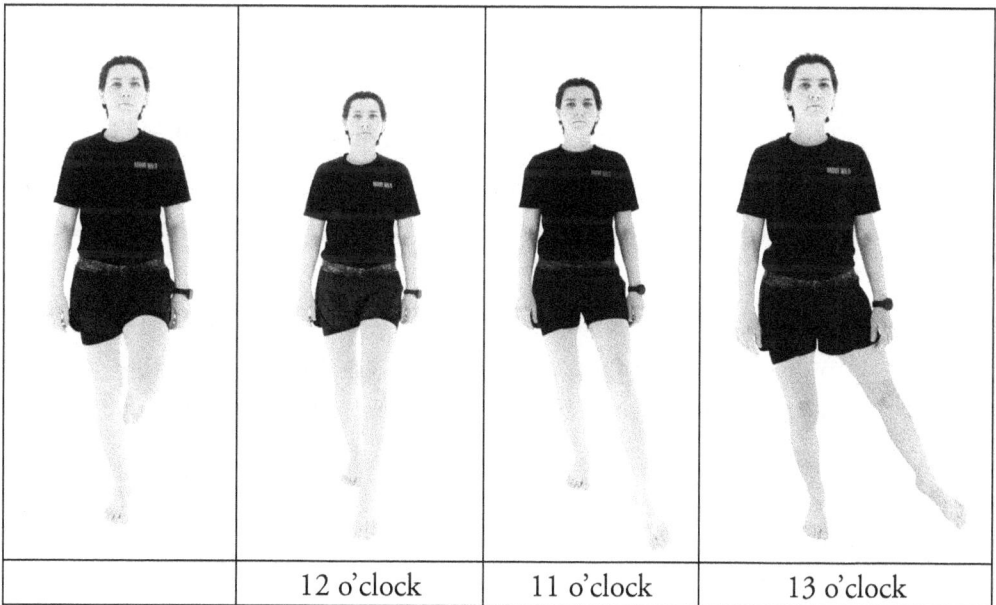

	12 o'clock	11 o'clock	13 o'clock

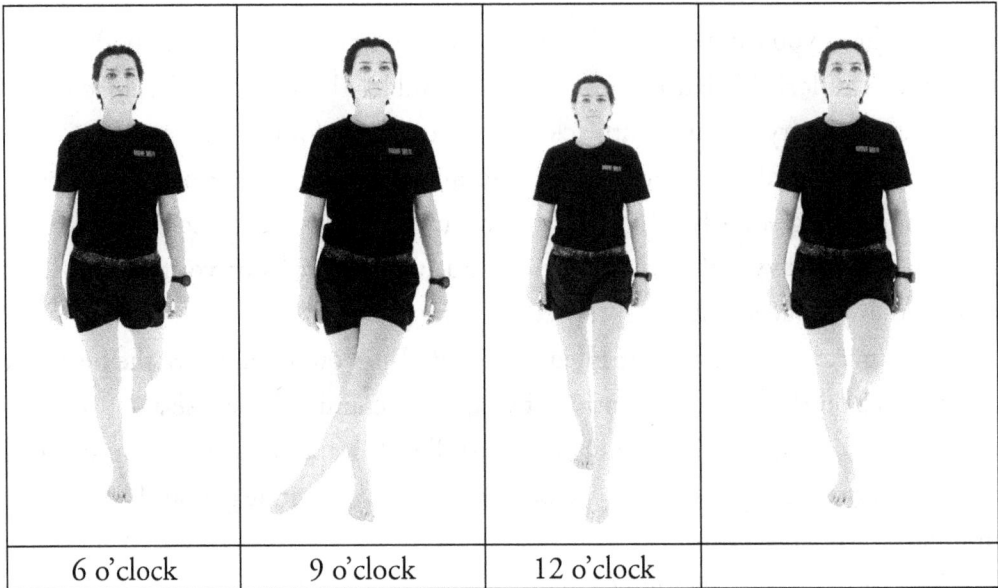

6 o'clock	9 o'clock	12 o'clock	

The Clock, all the way round

When you balance on your left leg, you go clockwise, 12, 1, 2, 3...9 (behind the left leg) and 10, 11 and 12 in front of the left leg.

Breathe normally throughout the exercise, while relaxing your shoulders, arms and hands. Ensure that your hips are aligned. It is essential that the hips don't go out of alignment. Performing this exercise correctly can strengthen the stability muscles and prevent joints from going out of alignment, so ultimately it can help reduce the risk of early wear and tear. This is especially important for runners as when we run we constantly balance on one leg. If the hips fall out of alignments a few thousand times (with every step) during every run, wear and tear can creep in and so can injuries.

Common errors and/or weaknesses to be aware of:

- Transferring body weight onto the balls of the feet. The heel should be nailed into the ground and stable throughout.

- Leaning back, forwards or to the side when reaching out around the clock. Keep alignment or think about realigning the 3 elements: nose-solar plexus-belly button. (see *The Clock, common mistakes*)
- Hips go out of alignment, pushing towards the outside. In this case the nose-solar plexus-belly button are not on top of each other anymore. Tuck in or tense the buttock on the corresponding side to bring everything back into alignment (see *The Clock, common mistakes*).
- Support knee collapsing in. The knee should track the toes as much as possible (see *The Clock, common mistakes*).
- Toes turn and point outwards. This can lead to over pronation of the foot and the knee buckling, followed by the hip. The outside of the foot should point forward and the toes slightly to the inside (see *The Clock, common mistakes*).

Leaning backwards to reach forward. Maintain your alignment.	Leaning forward to reach backwards. This can also be caused by tight hip flexors. Reach as far as you can while maintaining alignment.	Hip is out alignment.

Support foot turning out. Try to keep your toes facing forward.	Support knee buckling. Ensure your knee is in line with your toes.	

The Clock common mistakes

Depending on your fitness level you can go round the clock and back.

However, when technique is lost, change legs and then come back and resume where you left off.

Another option is to go around a quarter of the clock or half with a very correct technique and keep changing legs. You could balance on the left leg for a quarter, balance on the right leg for a quarter, balance on the left leg for another quarter, balance on the right leg for another quarter and so on.

This exercise is about how slowly and with how much control you can move, not about how much you can do or how far you can stretch. You have to judge when it is time to stop, take a break or change legs. The priority is to keep the form. In order of importance:

1. Keep your form.
2. Move slowly.

3. Reach far, without compromising on alignment.

4. As you get better, keep going for a longer time without putting the foot down.

360 DEGREES

The 360 Degrees balance exercise is similar to the Clock. However, instead of pointing the foot to each number around the clock and coming back into the Crane, you go round the clock in a circle, all the way round and back round, without returning to the Crane.

Benefits

Like the Clock, the 360 Degrees exercise is excellent for strengthening your foot, ankle, knee and hip stability muscles. These are essential when trying to correct certain imbalances, as when performing slow movements, all weaknesses and imbalances come to light. When performed correctly this exercise can address and correct some of these imbalances, if not all.

It also strengthens the quads, adductors, abductors and gluteus muscles, which it turn stabilise the hips and knees.

It obviously improves balance, as well as posture, postural awareness and focus. This can help in situations when you would use your balance. You will be more likely to be able to swiftly recover your balance or even control your fall. Good balance is essential to movement.

To maintain balance you should focus on also using your core muscles. Thus the core is working as well.

This exercise can reduce the risk of injuries such as ankle sprains or knee pain by strengthening stability muscles and mobilising the joints.

It can potentially speed up recovery from injury by strengthening stability muscles and correcting subtle imbalances as well as mobilising the joints.

Technical points

Begin by aligning the body – feet hip width apart, outsides of the feet pointing forwards, toes slightly inwards, knees soft, tail bone slightly tucked in, ears aligned with the shoulders, aligned with the hips, aligned with the ankles. Elongate the spine and relax your shoulders, arms and hands.

Imagine you are the centre of a clock. Distribute your bodyweight evenly on both feet and between the front (ball of foot and toes) and back (heel) of each foot.

Transfer your bodyweight onto the right foot and lift your left foot off the ground in the Crane position.

Bend your support leg slightly and ensure that the tripod is rooted into the ground. Activate your abdominal muscles and tense the right buttock so the right hip doesn't push out to the side, going out of alignment, and both hips are level. Keep elongating the body and looking forwards while the nose, solar plexus and belly button are connected by a straight line, stacked on top of each other (i.e. do not lean back, forwards or to the side).

Imagining you are the centre of a clock, point your left foot at 3 o'clock(behind or in front of your support leg). Do so without placing any weight at all on your left foot and while keeping the body in alignment.

Slowly and smoothly move your left foot in a circle around your body (clockwise or counter clockwise depending on whether you started with the left foot in front or behind the support foot) forming a uniform full circle by gently brushing the surface of the floor or ground as you go along. Your support leg can be straight or bent.

360 Degrees shows the exercise performed with the left leg, going from 3 o'clock front to 3 o'clock behind and back to 3 o'clock in front, so two full clocks. Here the left foot begins in front of the right foot, so it will go counter clockwise and then clockwise coming back.

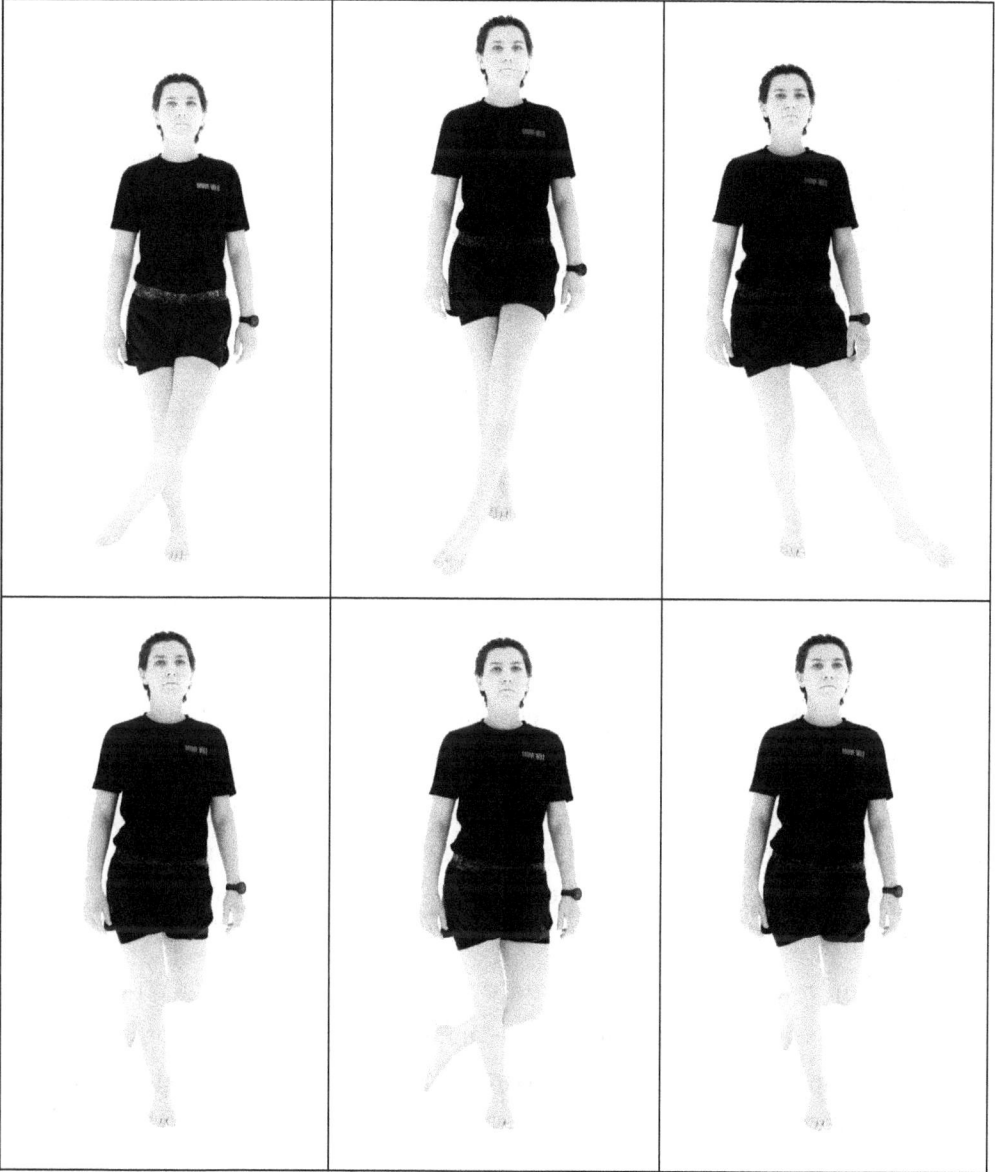

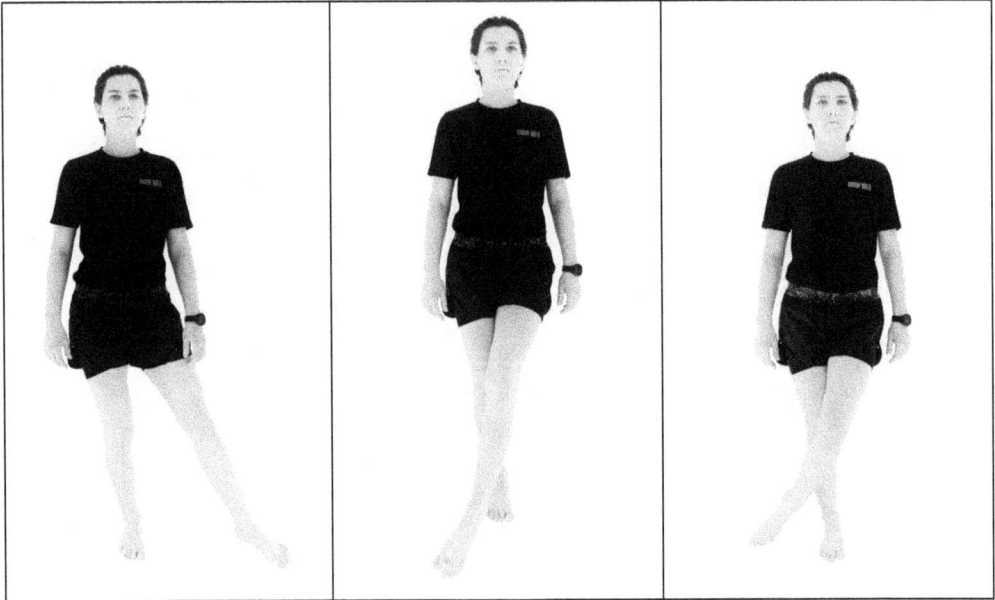

360 Degrees

Ensure that as you move along, you keep the tripod firmly rooted into the ground and the buttocks tensed.

Go all the way round the clock, until you reach 3 o'clock again, your start point. Reach as far as you can without changing your posture or your tripod or losing balance. Keep your body straight, with your core muscles engaged (belly button pulled in towards the spine).

Once you've done a full circle you can either change legs or repeat on the same leg. Just remember what you do on one side to repeat on the other. Breathe normally throughout the exercise, relaxing your shoulders, arms and hands.

Common errors and/or weaknesses to be aware of:

Similar to the Clock, you might be:

- Transferring body weight onto the balls of the feet. The heel should be nailed into the ground and stable throughout.

136

- Leaning back, forwards or to the side when reaching out round the clock. Keep alignment or think about realigning the 3 elements: nose-solar plexus-belly button (see *The Clock, common mistakes*).
- Hips go out of alignment, pushing towards the outside. In this case the nose-solar plexus-belly button are not on top of each other anymore. Tuck in or tense the buttock on the corresponding side to bring everything back in alignment (see *The Clock, common mistakes*).
- Support knee buckling. Knee should track the toes as much as possible (see *The Clock, common mistakes*).
- Toes turn and point outwards. This can lead to over pronation of the foot and the knee buckling, followed by the hip. The outside of the foot should point forward and the toes slightly to the inside (see *The Clock, common mistakes*).

Similar to the Clock

Depending on the fitness level you can go round the clock and back.

However when technique is lost or muscles hurt too much change legs and then come back and resume after a few minutes.

Another option is to go round a quarter or half with a very correct technique and keep changing legs. For instance, balance on the left leg for a quarter, balance on the right leg for a quarter, balance on the left leg for another quarter, balance on the right leg for another quarter and so on.

This exercise is about how slowly and with how much control you can move, not about how much you can do or how far you can stretch. You have to judge when it is time to stop, take a break or change legs. The priority is to keep the form. In order of importance:

1. Keep the form
2. Move very slowly
3. Reach far
4. Keep going for a long time

SEESAW

For this exercise you will need a small stick, pen or pencil and more space around you than the previous balance exercises required. You will be using the Seesaw method to place the stick or pen on the floor and then pick it up.

Benefits

This exercise aids understanding of balance and counterbalance, which can be useful in a diverse range of situations, such as when you lose balance or slip. With practice this becomes a reflex and, when required, the body can react instinctively and counterbalance to stabilise you or control your fall, which can sometimes be a better option than trying to recover your balance.

In line with the previous balance exercises, the Seesaw contributes by strengthening your foot, ankle, knee and hip stability muscles. These are essential when trying to correct certain imbalances, as when performing slow movements, all weaknesses and imbalances come to light. When performed correctly this exercise can address and correct some of these imbalances, if not all.

It also strengthens the quads, adductors, abductors and gluteus muscles, which it turn stabilise the hips and knees.

It obviously improves balance, as well as posture, postural awareness and focus. This can help in situations when you use your balance. You will be more likely to be able to swiftly recover your balance or even control your fall. Good balance is essential to movement.

To maintain balance you should focus on also using your core muscles. Thus the core is working as well.

This exercise can reduce the risk of injuries such as ankle sprains or knee pain by strengthening stability muscles and mobilising the joints.

It can potentially speed up recovery from injury by strengthening stability muscles and correcting subtle imbalances as well as mobilising the joints.

Technical points

Begin by aligning the body – feet hip width apart, outsides of the feet pointing forwards, toes slightly inwards, knees soft, tail bone slightly tucked in, ears aligned with the shoulders, aligned with the hips aligned with the ankles, elongating the spine and relaxing your shoulders, arms and hands.

Transfer your bodyweight on the right foot and lift your left foot off the ground. You should now be in the Crane position.

Bend your support leg slightly and ensure the tripod is rooted into the ground. Activate your abdominal muscles and tense the right buttock so the right hip doesn't push out to the side, going out of alignment, and both hips are level. Keep elongating the body and looking forwards while the nose, solar plexus and belly button are connected by a straight line, or think about them being stacked on top of each other (i.e. do not lean back, forwards or to the side).

Hold a stick/pen/pencil in your right hand. Keeping your back straight and chest proud, gently, through a slow, continuous movement, lower your upper body and lift the left leg behind you to counterbalance. When you're as low as you can go while keeping an excellent balance, place the stick on the ground as far from you as you can, again while maintaining balance. Don't stretch too far out, just place the stick as far away as you can.

Leave the stick on the ground and lift your upper body while lowering the leg behind you. Return in to the Crane position.

Throughout the movement, try to keep your back as straight as possible and both hips on the same line (i.e.do not lift the hip).

The Seesaw shows the full movement from the start position, the Crane, placing the stick on the ground and returning to the Crane.

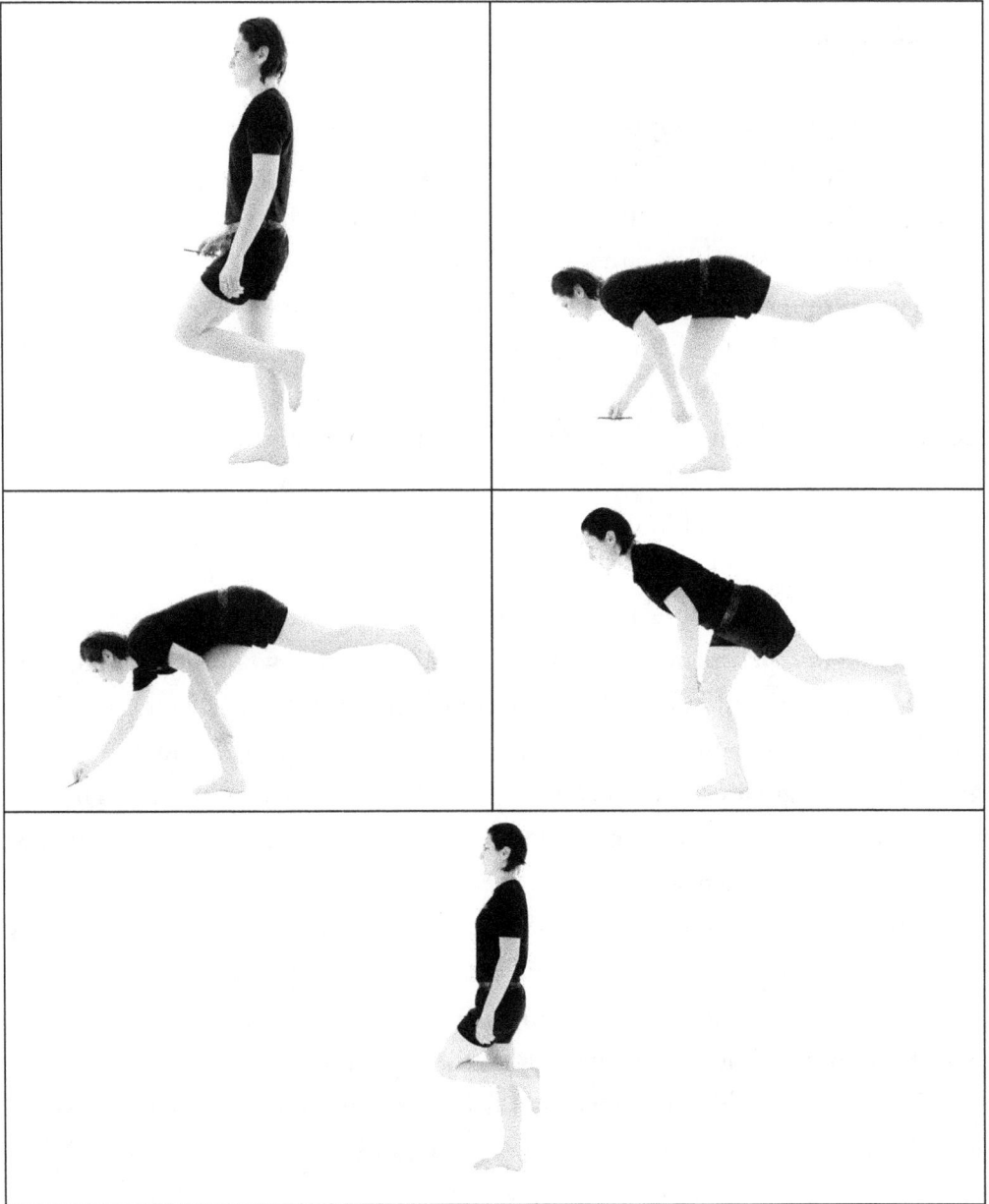

Seesaw

Try to keep an almost straight line at the hip (around the hip flexor area) as much as possible. Just like a seesaw, when one side goes down, the other side goes up almost in the same time (see *Seesaw diagram* and *Seesaw alignment*).

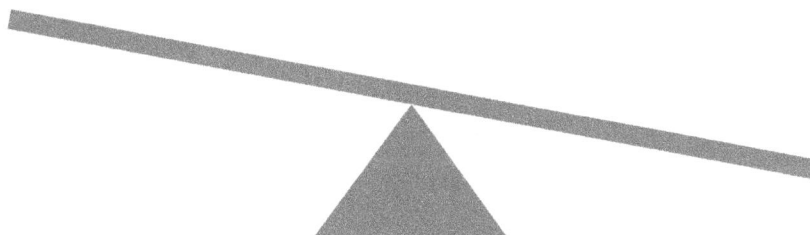

Seesaw diagram

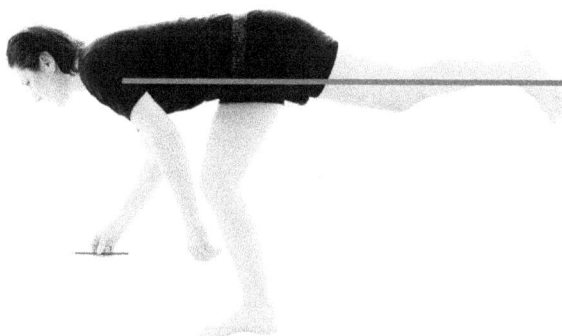

Seesaw alignment

Now you have to pick up the stick. After you return to the start position, the Crane, you can change legs or balance on the same leg and, following the same steps, pick up the stick.

Breathe normally throughout the exercise, and relax your shoulders, arms and hands when not in use. Remember to keep your back straight while activating the abdominal muscles.

Get creative with your body positioning and where you place the stick on the ground. Here are some ideas of changes to make each time you place the stick on the ground and/or each time you pick it up:

- change hands.
- change legs.
- change the angle at which you place the stick around you; use the numbers of the clock to place the stick at 12, 1, 2, 3 o'clock and so on.

141

- place it down with one hand and pick it up with the other, without changing legs, then change legs.
- place it down with your right/left hand to your right/left side and pick it up with your left/right hand, without changing legs, then change legs.

Come up with your own combinations. Have a look at *Seesaw variations* to get a visual representation of a couple of variations.

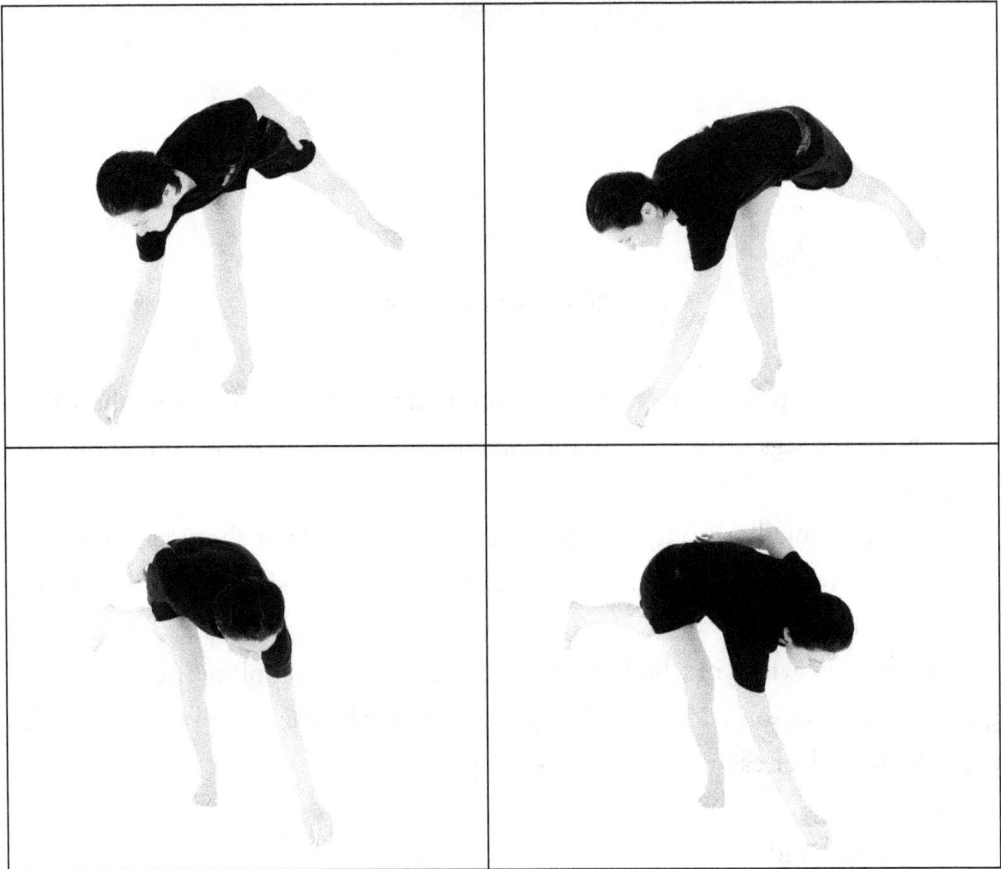

Seesaw variations

Common errors and/or weaknesses to be aware of:

- Hunching your upper and lower back before it's needed, that is at the end of the movement when placing the stick on the floor. Straighten the back, tense core muscles and lift the chest proud (see *Seesaw, errors*).
- Placing the stick too far away and then needing to alter the technique, shifting the weight on your toes and losing balance when you go to pick it up.
- Back leg is not coming up while the trunk is going down. There should be a straight line at the hip, or as close as possible. See *Seesaw alignment* for the correct form *and Seesaw, errors* for the errors.
- Transferring your body weight onto the balls of the feet. The tripod is not firmly rooted.
- Hips go out of alignment, pushing towards the outside. You can check this because the nose-solar plexus-belly button are not aligned anymore. Tuck in or tense the buttock on the corresponding side to bring everything back into alignment.
- Support knee is buckling. The knee should track the toes. See *Seesaw, errors*.
- Support foot points out. This can lead to over pronation of the foot and the knee buckling, followed by the hip. The outside of the foot should point forwards and the toes slightly to the inside. See *Seesaw, errors*.

Back bent and leg not lifting to counter balance.	Support foot turning out.	Knee buckling

Seesaw, errors

PRONE BODYWEIGHT TRANSFER

Prepare for a 7-stage balance and bodyweight transfer. This exercise is performed while in the Panther position. So grab yourself a mat or find your favourite fluffy carpet and let's begin.

Benefits

Since this is a balance and bodyweight exercise, the benefits are very similar to the previous exercises of the same type. However, I would add that here you work much more with your core. When performed correctly, it s train the core's deepest layers as well as the spine's stability muscles.

This exercise helps to strengthen the foot, ankle, knee and hip stability muscles as well as the quads (much more than previous balance exercises), adductors, abductors and glutes which in turn stabilise the knees and hips.

It strengthens the upper body as your position is exclusively in a Panther walk position. It stabilises the shoulder joint and mobilises and strengthens wrists and ankles.

It helps to reduce the risk of injuries such as ankle sprains and knee injuries by strengthening and mobilising key areas of the body listed above. When injuries do happen, it contributes to a speedy recovery by strengthening and mobilising the area.

Technical points

Begin by aligning the body and elongating the spine. Just as you would in a Panther Walk, lower yourself into a full squat and then into a Panther Walk position. While holding the shoulders over the wrists, back straight, knees under the hips and abdominal muscles activated, perform the following sequences:

Stage 1 – Arms *(Prone BWT, arms)*

Keep the knee under the hips and as low as possible. Your wrists are under the shoulders and your abdominal muscles are activated.

Transfer the body weight onto your right arm and lift the left hand off the ground. Hold for 3–5 seconds. Place the left hand back on the ground.

Transfer the body weight on your left arm and lift the right hand off the ground. Hold for 3–5 seconds, before placing back down.

Ensure that there is minimal hip movement. Perform the movement 8–10 times on each side before moving to the next stage.

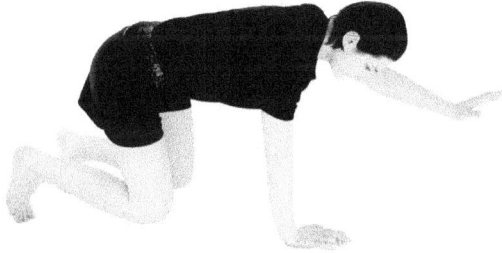

Prone BWT, arms

Stage 2 – Legs *(Prone BWT, legs)*

Keep the knees under the hips and as low as possible. Your wrists are under the shoulders and your abdominal muscles activated.

Transfer the body weight onto the left leg and lift the right foot off the ground. Hold for 3–5 seconds before placing it back down.

Transfer the body weight on the right leg and lift the left foot off the ground. Hold for 3–5 seconds before placing it back down

Ensure there is minimal hip movement. Perform the movement 8–10 times on each side before moving to the next stage.

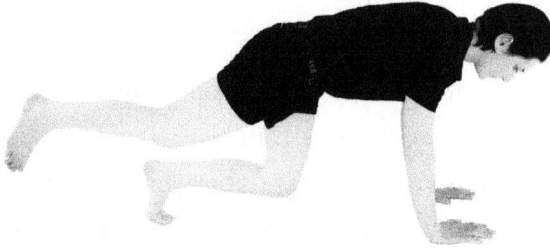

Prone BWT, legs

Progression:

- place a tennis ball on the lower back and try to perform the exercises without dropping the ball
- stretch out the arm/leg in front/behind as you lift each one in turn
- hold position for a longer time
- perform exercise on unstable surface or incline

Regression:

- just lift your hand and/or foot off the floor a few centimetres or inches
- lift and hold for less time

Stage 3 – Arm and opposite leg (*Prone BWT, arm and opposite leg*)

Keep the knees under the hips and as low as possible before and when lifting. Your wrists are under the shoulders and your abdominal muscles activated.

Lift the **left hand AND right foot** off the floor and hold for 3–5 seconds. Place them back down.

Lift the **right hand AND left foot.** Hold for 3–5 seconds and place back down.

Ensure there is minimal hip movement. Perform the movement 8–10 times before moving to the next stage.

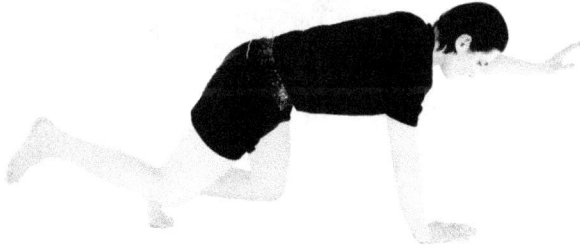

Prone BWT, arm and opposite leg

Progression:

- place a tennis ball on the lower back and try to perform the exercises without dropping the ball
- stretch out the arm/leg in front/behind as you lift them one by one
- hold position for a longer time
- perform exercise on unstable surface or incline

Regression:

- just lift your hand and/or foot off the floor a few centimetres or inches.
- hold position for less time
- go back to stages 1 and 2

Stage 4 – Connect under the body *(Prone BWT, connect under the body)*

Keep the knees under the hips and as low as possible before and when lifting. Your wrists are under the shoulders and your abdominal muscles activated.

Lift the **left arm AND right leg**. Connect them midway ***under*** your body and place them back down.

Change to the other side. Lift the **right arm AND left leg**. Connect them midway ***under*** your body and place them back down.

Ensure that there is minimal hip movement and that the movement is slow and fluid. Perform the movement 8–10 times before moving on to the next stage.

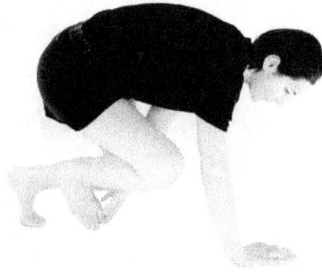

Prone BWT, connect under the body

Progression:

- perform the movements continuously for a number of times or seconds very slowly and with correct technique, without placing the hand and foot on the floor
- introduce deep breathing, breathing out when you bring the hand and leg in, breathing in when you extend
- extend the arm and leg out in front and behind respectively, like a half-superman position, before coming back in under the body or placing them back down
- hold the position under the body and/or stretched out for a few seconds
- perform the exercise on an unstable surface or incline

Regression:

- go back to stages 1, 2 and 3 until you master those and then return to stage 4.

Stage 5 – Connect over/behind the body *(Prone BWT, connect over/behind the body)*

Keep the knees under the hips and as low as possible before and when lifting. Your wrists are under the shoulders and your abdominal muscles activated.

Lift the **left arm AND right leg**. Connect them midway **_over/behind_** your body and place them back down.

Change on the other side. Lift the **right arm AND left leg**. Connect them mid way *over/behind* your body and place them back down.

Ensure there is minimal hip movement and the movement is slow and fluid. Perform the movement 8–10 times before moving onto the next stage.

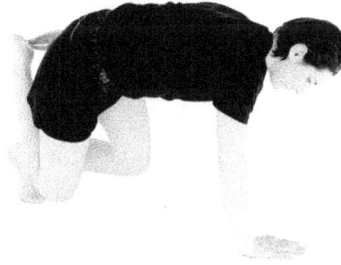

Prone BWT, connect over/behind the body

Progression:

- perform the movements continuously for a number of times or seconds very slowly and with correct technique, without placing the hand and foot on the floor
- hold the end position for a few seconds
- perform the exercise on an unstable surface or incline

Regression:

- go back to the previous stages and master those first

Stage 6 – Connect under and over the body in one movement

Now we bring Stages 4 and 5 together in one movement. Keep the knees under the hips and as low as possible before and when lifting. Your wrists are under the shoulders and your abdominal muscles activated.

Lift the **right arm AND left leg** and connect them **under and then over/ behind** your body straight away, without placing the foot or hand on the floor. Then place them back on the floor.

Change sides and perform the same movement with the left arm and right leg.

Ensure there is minimal hip movement and the movement is performed slow and fluid. Perform the movement 8–10 times before moving on to the next stage.

Progression:

- perform the movements continuously for a number of times or seconds very slowly and with correct technique, without placing the hand and foot on the floor
- hold position for a few seconds every time you connect hand with foot
- perform the exercise on an unstable surface or incline

Regression:

- go back to the previous stages and master those first

Stage 7 – Over and under the body

This is similar to Stage 6 but the other way around. Keep the knees under the hips and as low as possible before and when lifting. Your wrists are under the shoulders and your abdominal muscles activated.

Lift the **right arm AND left leg** and connect them **over and then under** your body straight away, without placing the foot or hand on the floor.

Change sides and perform the same movement with the left arm and right leg.

Ensure there is minimal hip movement and the movement is slow and fluid. Perform the movement 8–10 times.

Progression:

- perform the movements continuously for a number of times or seconds very slow and with correct technique, without placing the hand and foot on the floor
- hold position for a few seconds every time you connect hand with foot
- perform the exercise on an unstable surface or incline

Regression:

- go back to the previous stages and master those first

Common errors and/or weaknesses to be aware of:

- Hunching over. As with the Panther Walk position the back should be kept in a neutral alignment as much as possible and when appropriate. There is some movement, but it is not exaggerated.
- Lifting one hip. This is normal, especially with beginners until the stability muscles strengthen and the body adapts to this type of exercise. Keep the knees close to the ground, and the core tensed and the hips will also stay aligned.
- Transferring too much of the body weight onto the arms or legs. Body weight should be distributed evenly on arms and legs as much as possible, as with the Panther Walk. When there is only one hand and two feet on the ground, the legs take more weight and vice versa.
- Lifting the support knee too high. Keep the support knee as low as possible without touching the ground. If that's not yet possible stay focused on this element until you get stronger.
- If the support knee hurts, check whether there is too much weight on it. Alternatively go back and practise the fundamental balance exercises to strengthen the stability muscles.

Review the basic errors and correction on the Panther Walk as there are similar elements.

SUPINE BODYWEIGHT TRANSFER

A second seven stage exercise, similar to the previous one, is performed from a Crab Walk position which you should be familiar with by now.

Benefits

On top of the balance and bodyweight transfer benefits, the particular benefit of this exercise comes from its position. It is particularly beneficial for mobility of the wrists, shoulders and hips. Furthermore, when performed with good form, it's really good for postural improvement as it stretches the pectorals (chest muscles) as well as the shoulders.

It is also a good exercise for upper body strength and toning in general, particularly shoulders and triceps.

As with every Move Wild exercise, it trains the core as well. And let's not forget the glutes, if you hold your hips high and don't let them move from side to side when transferring the bodyweight.

Technical points

Begin by aligning the body and elongating the spine. Lower yourself into a full squat and then place yourself in a Crab Walk position. While holding the shoulders over the wrists, hips high above the ground, buttocks tensed, fingers pointing the same way as the toes and head out of the shoulders (make more space between your ears and your shoulders) perform the following sequences:

Stage 1 – Arms

Transfer the body weight onto the left arm and lift the right hand. Hold for 3–5 seconds and place it back down.

Transfer the body weight onto your right arm and lift the left hand off the ground. Hold for 3–5 seconds and place it back down.

Ensure that there is minimal hip movement, you don't drop your hips and the movement is performed slowly and in a fluid manner. Perform the movement 8–10 times in total before moving on to the next stage.

Keep your head out of the shoulders and look forwards. Your support wrist is under the shoulder, hips are off the ground, as high as you can get them, and your abdominal muscles are activated. The glutes are activated as well.

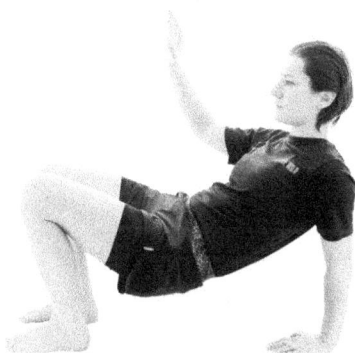

Supine BWT, arms

Stage 2 – Legs

Transfer the body weight onto the right leg and lift the left foot off the ground. Hold for 3–5 seconds and place it back down.

Transfer the body weight onto the left leg and lift the right foot. Hold for 3–5 seconds and place it back down.

Ensure that there is minimal hip movement, you don't drop your hips and the movement is performed slowly and in a fluid manner. Perform the movement 8–10 times in total before moving on to the next stage.

Keep your head out of the shoulders and look forwards. Your wrists are under the shoulders, hips are off the ground, as high as you can get them, and your abdominal muscles are activated. The glutes are activated as well, especially the support leg side.

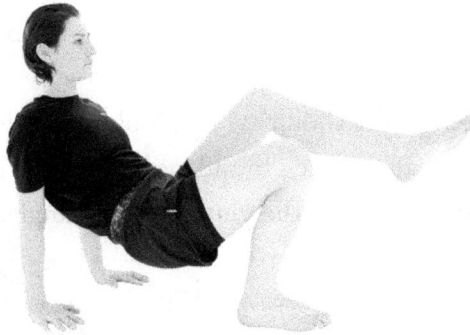

Supine BWT, legs

Progression:

- stretch out the arms and legs as you lift them one by one
- hold arm/leg stretched out for a longer time
- lift hips higher

Regression:

- just lift your hand off the floor a few centimetres or inches, rather than all the way up
- just transfer as much of the body weight as possible onto the other 3 limbs and hold, without lifting the hand or foot off the ground

Stage 3 – Arm and opposite leg

Keep your head out of the shoulders and look forwards. Your support wrist is under the shoulder, hips are off the ground, as high as you can get them, and your abdominal muscles are activated. The glutes are activated as well, especially on the support leg side.

Lift the **left hand and right foot,** hold for 3–5 seconds and place them back down.

Lift the **right hand and left foot,** hold for 3–5 seconds.

Ensure that there is minimal hip movement, you don't drop your hips and the movement is performed slowly and in a fluid manner. Perform the movement 8–10 times before moving on to the next stage.

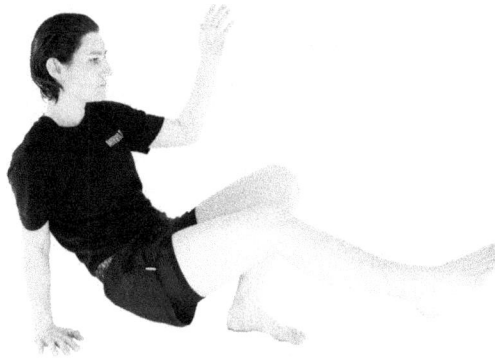

Supine BWT, arm and opposite leg

Progression:

- stretch out the arm and leg as you lift them one by one
- lift arm and leg on the same side (i.e. left arm and left leg)
- hold stretched out position for longer
- lift hips higher

Regression:

- just lift off the floor a few centimetres or inches
- go back to stages 1 and 2

Stage 4 – Connect over/in front of the body

Keep your head out of the shoulders and look forwards. Your support wrist is under the shoulder, hips are off the ground, as high as you can get them, and your abdominal muscles are activated. The glutes are activated as well, especially the support leg side.

Lift the **left hand and right foot.** Bring them together over the body, or in front of you. Once you connect them, place them back down. You can also hold this position if you wish.

Lift the **right hand and left foot.** Bring them together over the body and place them back down.

Ensure that there is minimal hip movement, you don't drop your hips and the movement is performed slowly and in a fluid manner. Perform the movement 8–10 times before moving on to the next stage.

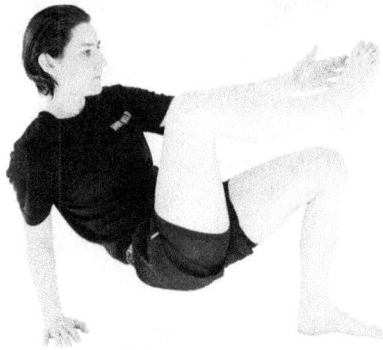

Supine BWT, connect over/in front of the body

Progression:

- perform the movements continuously for a number of times or seconds very slowly and with correct technique, without placing the hand and foot on the floor
- introduce deep breathing, breathing out when you bring the hand and leg together (when you "compress" your body you squeeze air out and tense your abs), breathing in when you extend
- hold the position over the body for a few seconds
- perform the exercise on an unstable surface or incline

Regression:

- go back to stages 1, 2 and 3 until you master those and return to stage 4

Stage 5 – Connect under the body

Keep your head out of the shoulders and look forwards. Your support wrist is under the shoulder, hips are off the ground, as high as you can get them, and your abdominal muscles are activated. The glutes are activated as well, especially the support leg side.

Lift the **right hand and left foot.** Connect them under the body, through the gap between the leg and the body. Think of threading the leg through that gap.

Lift the **left hand and right foot** and perform the same movement.

Ensure that there is minimal hip movement, you don't drop your hips and the movement is performed slowly and in a fluid manner. Perform the movement 8–10 times before moving on to the next stage.

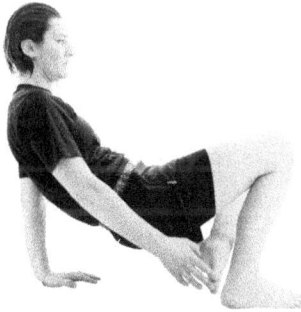

Supine BWT, connect under the body

Progression:

- perform the movements continuously for a number of times or seconds very slowly and with correct technique, without placing the hand and foot on the floor

- introduce deep breathing, breathing out when you bring the hand and leg together (when you "compress" your body you squeeze air out and tense your abs), breathing in when you extend
- hold the position over the body for a few seconds
- perform the exercise on an unstable surface or incline

Regression:

- go back to stages 1, 2 and 3 until you master those

Stage 6 – Connect over and under the body

Bring Stages 4 and 5 together in one movement.

Lift the **left arm and right leg** and connect them over and then under the body straight away, without placing the foot or hand on the floor.

Perform the same movement with the **right arm and left leg.**

Keep your head out of the shoulders and look forwards. Your support wrist is under the shoulder, hips are off the ground, as high as you can get them, and your abdominal muscles are activated. The glutes are activated as well, especially the support leg side.

Ensure that there is minimal hip movement, you don't drop your hips and the movement is performed slowly and in a fluid manner. Perform the movement 8–10 times before moving on to the next stage.

Progression:

- perform the movements continuously for a number of times or seconds very slowly and with correct technique, without placing the hand and foot on the floor
- introduce deep breathing
- hold the position over the body for a few seconds
- perform the exercise on an unstable surface or incline

Regression:

- go back to stages 1, 2 and 3 until you master those

Stage 7 – Connect under and over the body

This is similar to Stage 6 but in reverse.

Lift the **left arm and right leg** and connect them under and then over the body straight away, without placing the foot or hand on the floor.

Perform the same movement with the **right arm and left leg.**

Keep your head out of the shoulders and look forwards. Your support wrist is under the shoulder, hips are off the ground, as high as you can get them, and your abdominal muscles are activated. The glutes are activated as well, especially the support leg side.

Ensure that there is minimal hip movement, you don't drop your hips and the movement is performed slowly and in a fluid manner. Perform the movement 8–10 times.

Progression:

- perform the movements continuously for a number of times or seconds very slowly and with correct technique, without placing the hand and foot on the floor
- introduce deep breathing
- hold the position over the body for a few seconds
- perform the exercise on an unstable surface or incline

Regression:

- go back to stages 1, 2 and 3 until you master those

Common errors to be aware of:

The errors to be aware of are similar the the ones in the Crab Walk.

- Head sinking into the shoulders. As with the Crab Walk, the neck should be lengthened and shoulders stabilised, with lats (latissimus dorsi muscles on your back which extend to the sides of the body) activated. Make space between the ears and the shoulders.
- Hips are too low and you don't get the benefits of the exercise.
- Not transferring the body weight before attempting to lift the limbs off the ground. To be able to lift a part of the body, 100% of the weight has to be carried by the other parts of the body to "unlock" the one you want to lift. It makes sense, yet a lot of people don't do it.

It is very important to remember to lengthen the head out of the shoulders (i.e. make space between the ears and the shoulders). This activates the lats, stabilises the shoulder joints and avoids shoulder injuries.

Go back to the Crab Walk and go through the fundamental points of the basic stance.

PRONE TO SUPINE FLOW

This movement takes place in the transverse plane and it's a switch from the prone or face-down position (Panther Walk) to the supine or face-up position (Crab Walk). It combines the Prone and Supine Body Weight Transfer movements. The only added element is the flow from one to another.

This is one way to switch from one position to the other, and it's an excellent exercise to mobilise the upper and lower back. For the purpose of learning from a book, the process is broken down into 3 steps. But first let's have a look at the benefits of the exercise.

Benefits

An excellent exercise which mobilises the hips and spine (lumbar and thoracic). It helps relieve tightness and soreness in the back. I would not recommend you to jump straight into this exercise if your back is sore; begin with the previous exercises.

It strengthens the foot, ankle, knee and hip stability muscles and the upper body in general, including the core.

It helps with stabilising, strengthening and mobilising the shoulder joints and mobilising and strengthening wrists and ankles.

It helps improve balance, posture and postural awareness and focus.

Technical points

Begin by aligning the body and elongating the spine. Lower yourself into a full squat and then into a Panther Walk position. This is your start position.

Stage 1:

Follow the pictures in *Prone to Supine Flow stage 1*. This is the flow from the Panther Walk to the Crab Walk position.

In the Panther Walk position, lift the left foot off the ground, keeping the support knee as close to the ground as you can, without touching the ground.

The left leg travels forwards and under the body, towards the right side. At the same time your body turns to face upwards. Another way to put it is threading the left leg under the body.

As you turn to face upwards, in a Crab Walk position, the right hand lifts off the floor and the left hand twists/pivots on the floor. The support foot, the right foot, also pivots on the spot.

Turn your whole body to face upwards in a Crab Walk position with the left foot and right hand off the floor. You can also place them on the floor if needed.

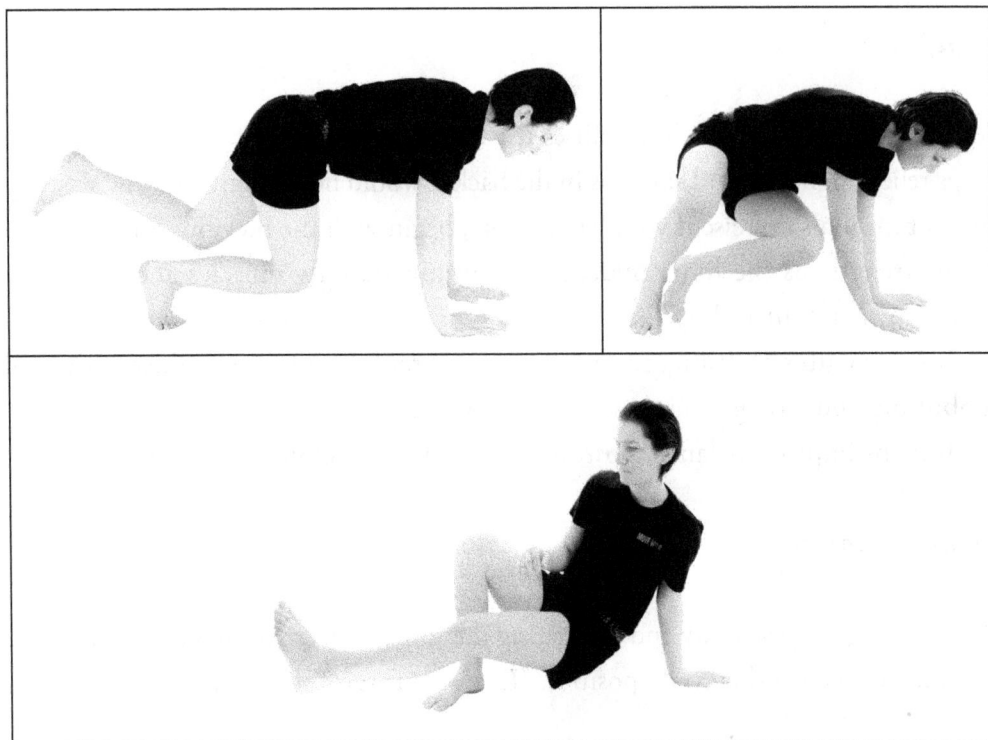

Prone to Supine Flow stage 1

Stage 2:

Follow the pictures from *Prone to Supine Flow stage 2*.

This is the flow back from Crab to Panther position via the same route, but in reverse.

Thread the left foot under the body, behind the right leg. Place the right hand back on the floor, pivot on the left hand and right foot and turn your body to face the ground.

As you turn, place the left foot on the floor (or you can also keep it up and ready to perform Stage 1 of the movement again).

Finish in a Panther Walk position with the left foot and right hand on or off the floor. This is the position you started in at Stage 1.

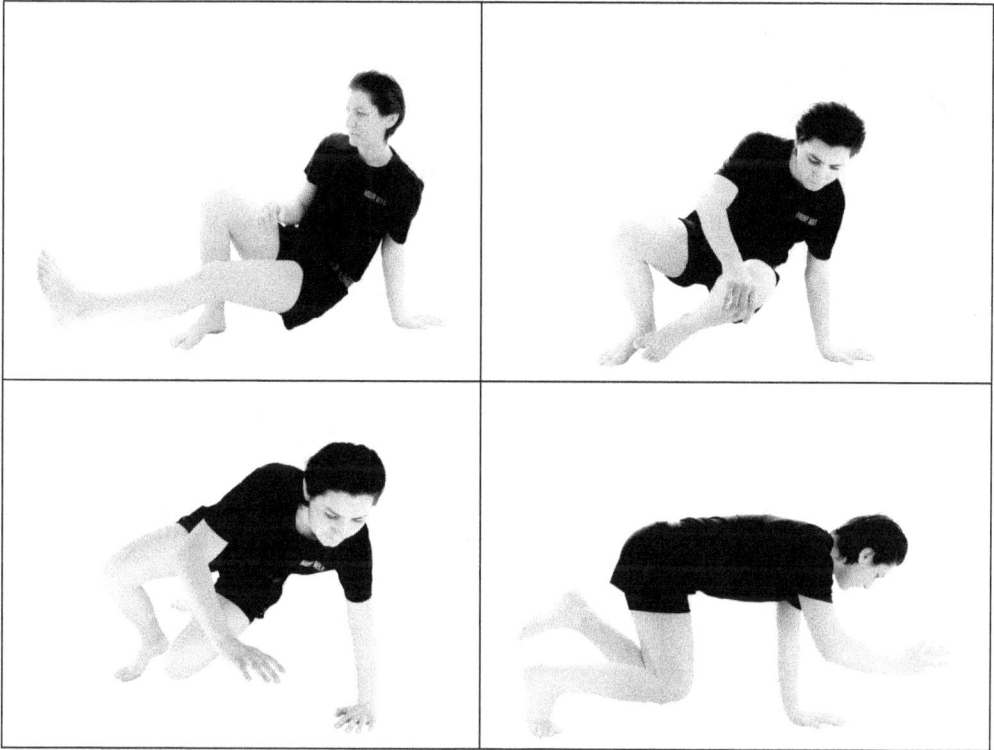

Prone to Supine Flow stage 2

You can now continue flowing back and forth as many times as you like. Make sure you perform the exercise on both sides.

Stage 3:

In stage 3 you don't stop to go back on the same route; instead you continue the movement.

Follow the pictures from *Prone to Supine Flow stage 3*.

Begin in a Crab Walk position. Thread the left leg underneath your body and finish in a Panther Walk position, as you did in stage 2. Now, instead of stopping in a Panther position, continue the movement over and around your body. Keep your hips as high as you can and land with your toes first, then the whole foot.

When the movement is finished you should be in a Crab Walk position. The foot that was in the air (left) now stays on the ground and the other foot (right) is up, ready to perform the same movement in the other direction.

Now your right leg is stretched out, threads under the body, goes over the top and lands on the ground in a Crab Walk position. You're back where you started from.

Prone to Supine Flow stage 3 shows the movement from both sides.

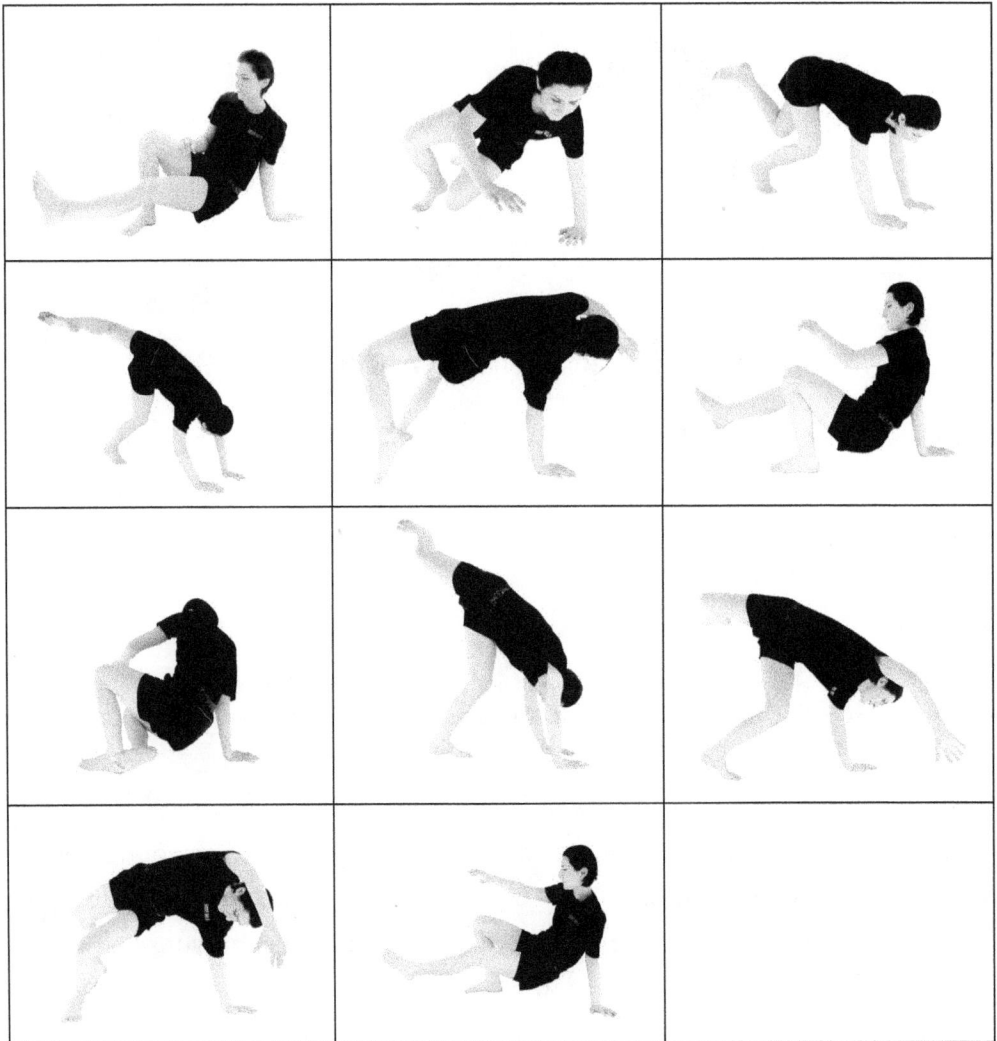

Prone-Supine Flow stage 3

As you land in your final Crab position ensure the bent leg is close to the body and the heel is on the ground.

Common errors and/or weaknesses to be aware of:

The following list addresses all three stages above.

- When the hips are too low in the Crab position there is no room for the foot and leg to move in and perform the flow; hips need to make room for the leg to pass through.
- The back should be kept in a neutral alignment as much as possible, particularly in the Panther position.
- Lifting the knee too high in the Panther position. Keep the knee as low as possible. This may not be possible straight away due to low strength. Staying focused on this element will slowly build the required strength. This way you get the most out of the exercise.
- Head sinking into the shoulders in the Crab position. As with the Crab Walk, the neck should be lengthened and the shoulders stabilised, with lats activated.
- At the end of the flow, when in the Crab Walk position, the support foot may be too far away from the body and/or the heel may be off the ground. The foot should be close to the body, almost under the hip and the whole foot should be on the ground. This allows you freedom of movement, control and balance.
- When performing the circular movement, the hips are very low. Strive to keep the hips as high as possible and be ready to touch the ground with the toes first, keeping the hips high. This helps you improve your mobility and balance among other benefits.

FLEXIBILITY AND MOBILITY

The Move Wild curriculum comprises four main stretching movements which stretch the major lower body muscles (i.e. quadriceps, hip flexors, hamstrings, adductors, abductors, gluteus). All Move Wild movements have a flexibility and mobility aspect, however, these 3 put the emphasis on stretching. From these four main stretching exercises, variations can be created. The four fundamental exercises are:

1. The Lizard
2. The Pigeon
3. The Side Kick Frog
4. The Gorilla

It is important to remember that the following pictures show the position you are aiming for. Don't stretch beyond your means just to position yourself as you see in the pictures. If the Move Wild flexibility exercises are too demanding at the moment, practise all the other Move Wild exercises as they strengthen and release the muscles gradually, then, after a few weeks, test the flexibility exercises.

Remember to watch the videos on www.movewildacademy.com/move-wild to get a better understanding of the exercises. Password is "duckwalk"

THE LIZARD

Benefits

The Lizard stretches the hips flexors of the back leg primarily, as well as the glutes and hamstrings of the front leg. It also mobilises the hips.

It improves coordination and agility, as well as ankle mobility in dorsiflexion, especially if the front foot points forwards. When you move you should do so by keeping the front foot facing forwards and with the heel on the ground for as long as you can.

This is the counter stretch to the Pigeon, which you will learn next.

Technical points:

Begin in a press-up position (abdominal muscles activated, wrists under the shoulders etc.) and step forwards with the right foot to the outside of the right hand. Keep the right heel on the ground and place it as far forwards as you can without injuring yourself.

If you can, align the right foot with the right hand and keep the heel on the ground. The left leg is almost straight and stretched out behind, without touching the ground with the knee (unless you need to).

Ensure that your back is straight and you look forwards.

Walk forwards with your hands (about 4 steps to make room for the back leg to step through) and step forward with the left foot. The left knee and foot land outside the left hand and are aligned (if possible) with the left hand. The left heel is on the ground.

As you step forwards ensure that the heel of the front foot stays on the ground for as long as possible, with the toes pointing forwards, before the heel lifts off the ground.

As you step forwards keep moving your hands, taking 4 or even 5 steps with the hands. The back leg needs a lot of room.

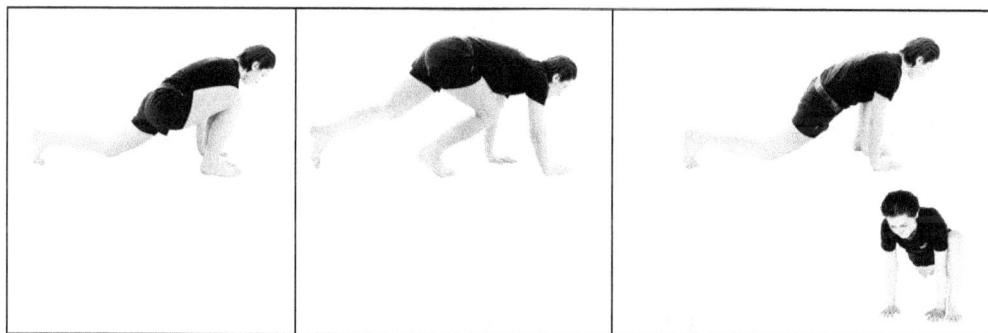

The Lizard

As you walk, keep your hips as low as you can throughout the movement and your front toes pointing forwards and walk with your hands as much as you need to make room for the back leg to come through.

Keep performing the Lizard and try to create an uninterrupted, fluid movement.

The Lizard can be used as a dynamic stretching exercise as well as a static stretch and can be performed forwards as well as backwards.

Common errors and/or weaknesses to be aware of:

- Not walking forwards enough with the hands, ending up with either the back leg too, the front heel off the ground and the hips high in the air or moving the back leg backwards to adjust the end position.
- Front heel comes off the ground while in the end position.
- Front toes/foot turn(s) out before stepping. This is a good ankle mobility exercise if the toes are pointed forwards and the heel stays on the ground for as long as possible. However, pay attention not to lift the hips too high while attempting to keep the heel on the ground.
- Hips come up too high so the stretch is reduced or not effective at all.

THE PIGEON

The Pigeon is an excellent hip mobility exercise as well as a stretch for the gluteus muscles. When done correctly it also lengthens the trunk and stretches the latissimus dorsi.

It is, however not suitable for people with knee injuries or pain. If you experience knee pain in general, skip over this movement.

Benefits

The Pigeon stretches the gluteus muscles primarily, and also stretches the hip flexors of the back leg.

It lightly stretches the upper and lower back and the latissimus dorsi.

It improves coordination, agility and ankle mobility in plantar flexion.

It certainly mobilises the hip joint and stretches the muscles all around it.

This is the counter stretch to the Lizard movement you learnt earlier, although the 2 movements overlap as they stretch similar muscles. The difference is that one emphasises hip flexor stretching and the other gluteus stretching.

Technical points

Begin in a press-up position and bring the left knee in between the hands, as far as you can. The foot is not quite under the body, but to the side.

Hips are levelled, with the buttocks off the ground. Avoid sitting down on one side. The upper body is straight and upright before leaning from the hips to reach forward. The back leg is stretched out behind you, relaxed, with the knee touching the ground. Point the back foot and toes.

To move, bend forwards from the hips, stretch out the arms in front of you and reach out with the hands as far as you can. Come up on the back knee and this time drive the right knee in between the hands.

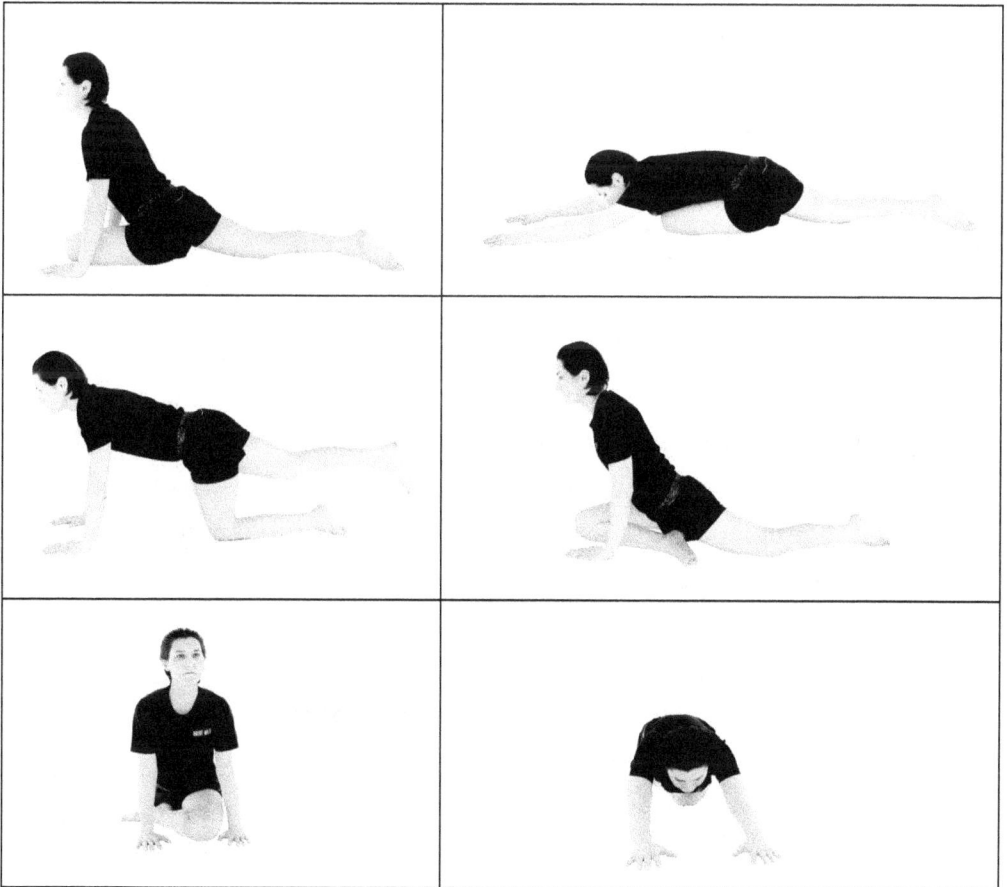

169

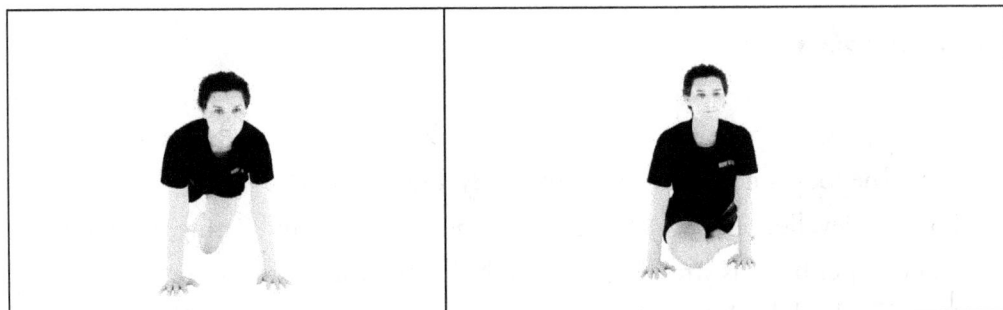

The Pigeon

The Pigeon shows the movement on one side only from two angles, moving from left leg forwards to right leg forwards. Continue the movement by bending forwards from the hips, stretching the arms out and reaching out with the hands as far as possible. Come up on the right knee and drive the left knee in between the hands.

Continue moving forwards with one leg and then the other, creating a smooth movement.

The Pigeon can be used as a dynamic stretching exercise as well as a static stretch and can be performed forwards as well as backwards.

Common errors and/or weaknesses to be aware of:

- Compressing the body. The upper body is either straight upwards or reaching and stretching forwards when moving, never compressed or hunched over.
- Sitting on one side of the buttocks, usually on the side with the bent leg. Ensure that the hips are level so you get the most out of the exercise.
- Front foot is under the body. Ensure the foot is out to the side as far as you can so you get the benefits of this exercise. If you don't feel a stretch on the glutes, it's probably because you are either sitting on the floor or your front foot is under the glutes.
- Not reaching far enough with the hands so the back knee doesn't have room to move forwards. This leads to either compressing the body or pushing the back leg backwards to lengthen and make room.

THE SIDE KICK FROG

The Side Kick Frog is an excellent stretch for the adductors and to really open up the hips. It is particularly strong on the hips, so warmup with the Lizard and Pigeon first if you decide to do the flexibility exercises and nothing else. And if you are a martial artist this is a great way to improve your side kick and general mobility and flexibility, hence the name.

Benefits

The Side Kick Frog is a movement that predominantly stretches the adductor muscles and improves hip mobility. It takes the joints through their full range of motion.

It develops coordination and agility, and improves ankle mobility.

Take care with this exercise as you can overstretch and pull a muscle if too much strain is applied. Begin with a thorough warmup and perform other movements before this one.

Technical points

Begin in a standing position and squat all the way down. Rock your body forwards and come up onto your toes, into the Frog Jump start position, with knees outside the arms.

In this example you will be moving towards the right side only. The photos are mirror images so move in the same direction as you look at the photos, I am moving to my left and your right.

Stretch the right leg to the side with toes pointing forwards and sole of foot on the floor. The left leg hasn't moved and is still under your body with the left knee outside the elbow.

Bend the right knee and transfer the bodyweight towards the right. Now your right leg is bent and your left leg is straight.

Shift your bodyweight onto your arms and, as you hop, shuffle the left foot under your body and stretch your right leg to the side, toes landing first. Now you are back with the right leg stretched out and the left leg under your body.

171

Continue towards the right doing exactly the same movement (i.e. shifting the body weight onto the right leg, shuffling the feet under the body, left leg moving in and right leg stretching out). Then do the same again, moving to the left.

The Side Kick Frog shows the full movement.

Keep your hips as low as possible as you transfer the body weight. In this exercise you don't lift off the ground too high as you would in the Frog Jump, you just hover as you switch or shuffle the legs under the body.

Try to step, or rather slide, into the end position with toes first, making the landing soft and controlled.

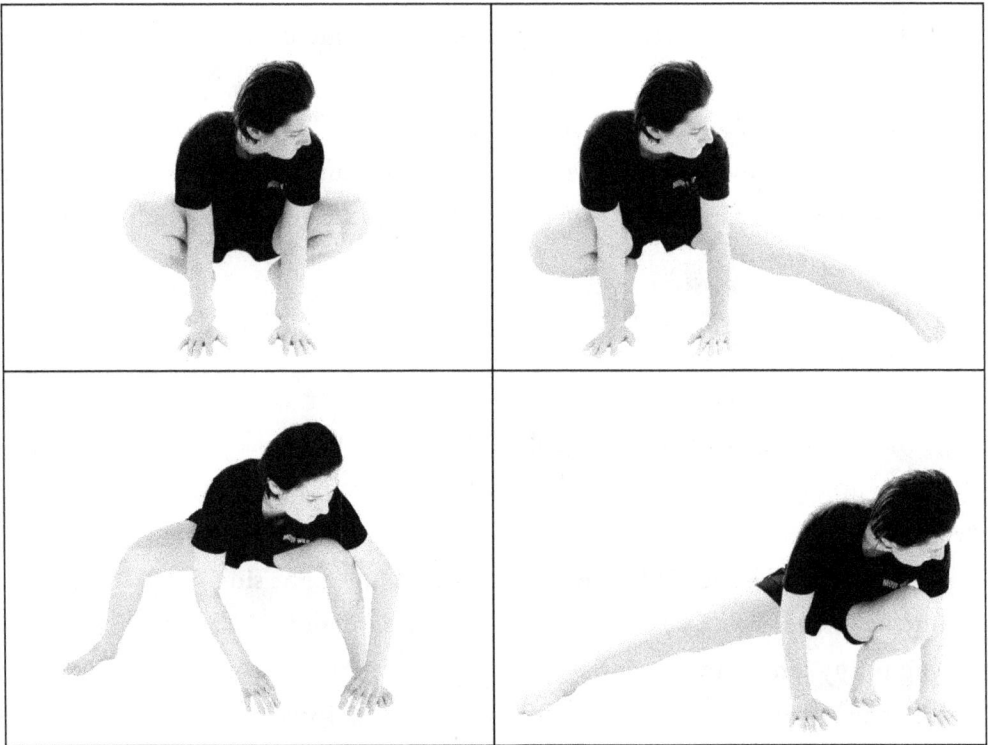

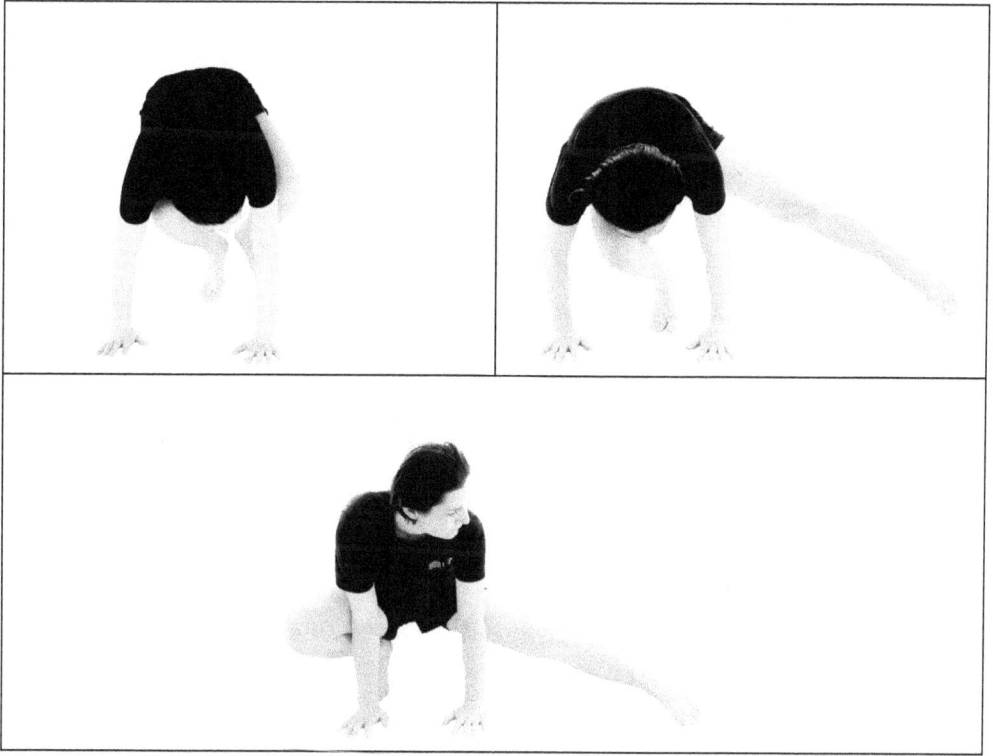

The Side Kick Frog

Regression: Instead of hopping and shuffling, just step in and out with your feet

Progression:

- Create a continuous movement, without stopping after each shuffle. Even when you move fast try to fully stretch out the legs and touch your heel with your buttocks before engaging in the next movement.
- Land with both feet at the same time
- Hold the position for a fraction of a second, or even a second, in the air, using your core, before landing

Common errors and/or weaknesses to be aware of:

- Lifting the outside of the foot off the floor on the stretched out leg. This is very important because, in that situation, the knee is in a compromised position, placing a lot of pressure on the outside of the knee. Do you best to keep the sole of foot flat on the floor all the time. Lifting the outside of the foot off the floor causes the knee to collapse inwards and place unnecessary pressure on it.
- Lifting hips too high when shifting your bodyweight from one side to the other. This is normal at the beginning while the joints and muscles open up and stretch. Once you have adjusted to the exercise, in order to get the most out of it opening up the hips and stretching the muscles, keep the hips as low as possible when transferring the bodyweight.
- Holding the hips high after the shuffle. After each shuffle you should end up in the starting position, with one leg stretched out and the other under the body, touching the heel with the buttocks (or as close as possible).
- Toes not pointing forwards. To stretch and also mobilise the ankles, try to keep the toes facing forwards as much you can, on both feet. You can point them out while you transfer the body weight. As with all the exercises it's important to acknowledge where there are challenges and adapt. If the toes can't point straight forwards just do your best to come as close as possible.
- The exercise is very tough on the hips, especially for someone who has never done this before. Take it slowly, step by step, performing other hip opening exercise beforehand, such as the other Frog exercises, Tiger, Lizard and Pigeon.
- People with knee pain might feel some pain when transferring the body from one side to the other. In this case pointing the toes outwards, as opposed to forwards, can help. However, pointing toes outwards too much may cause the knee to collapse inwards which can also affect the knee. Try variations, but, if the pain persists, change the exercise.

Variation:

Instead of the toes facing forwards with the sole of the foot on the floor, lift the toes upwards after landing. When transferring the bodyweight, point the toes and place the sole of the foot on the ground. Transfer the body weight and shuffle as usual. Remember to perform the exercise on both sides.

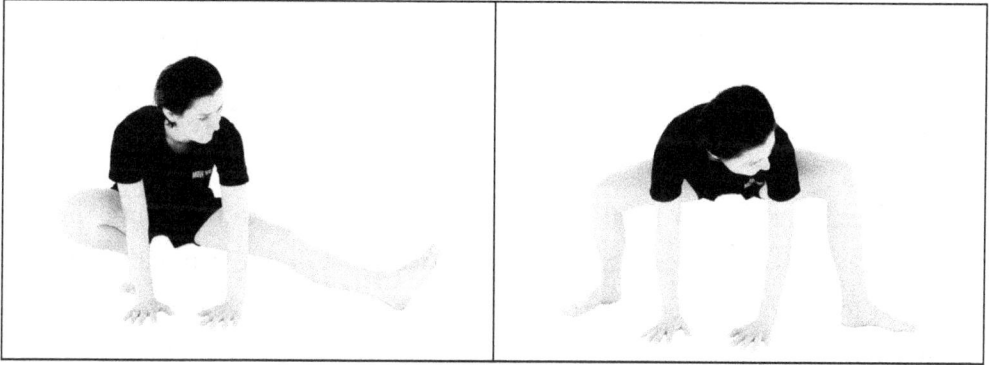

Side Kick Frog, variation

The regression of the variation is the same as for the original exercise, stepping instead of jumping.

THE GORILLA

The Gorilla is a great exercise to stretch the calves and hamstrings and, for those with a tight lower back, it also stretches this.

Benefits

The Gorilla stretches the back chain which comprises of the calves, hamstrings and back, while mobilising ankles in dorsiflexion and improving hip mobility.

Lastly, it also strengthens the core when the movement is performed with as little hip side movement as possible.

Take care, as hypotension might occur when standing up.

Technical points

Begin in a standing position, elongating the body, with toes pointing forwards and feet hip width apart. Keeping your legs as straight as you can, bend over from the hips, reach towards your toes and walk your hands forwards until your palms are fully on the ground.

You should now be an inverted V shape like so ∧, or as close as possible. If needed, allow your knees to bend and your heels to come off the ground. The aim is to gradually improve your mobility and flexibility so your legs are straight and heels on the ground. So begin where you can and work your way to the end goal from there.

Begin walking forwards, alternating hands and feet, and keeping the toes pointing forwards. If you can, step with your heels first, if not step with your toes. Step as far forwards as you can, as close to your hands as possible while keeping the legs straight. If the legs bend, take a shorter step. Don't worry about which hand goes with which foot, just walk.

The abdominal muscles activate as you use them to move your legs forwards, instead of hitching up the leg from the hip. Prevent the hips from swaying from side to side and look towards your knees. Drive your chest towards your knees as best you can and try to keep your back straight. Toes face forwards.

This movement can be performed backwards as well as forwards.

When you want to stop, reverse the steps: bring your hands towards your toes, place your heels on the ground and either uncurl your spine from the bottom to the top (buttocks tucked in and abdominal muscles tensed) or bend your knees, straighten your back and stand up through a squat. The point is to gradually come back to a standing position to avoid getting dizzy or injuring yourself due to jerky, uncontrolled movements.

Regression: step with the heel off the ground and legs bent

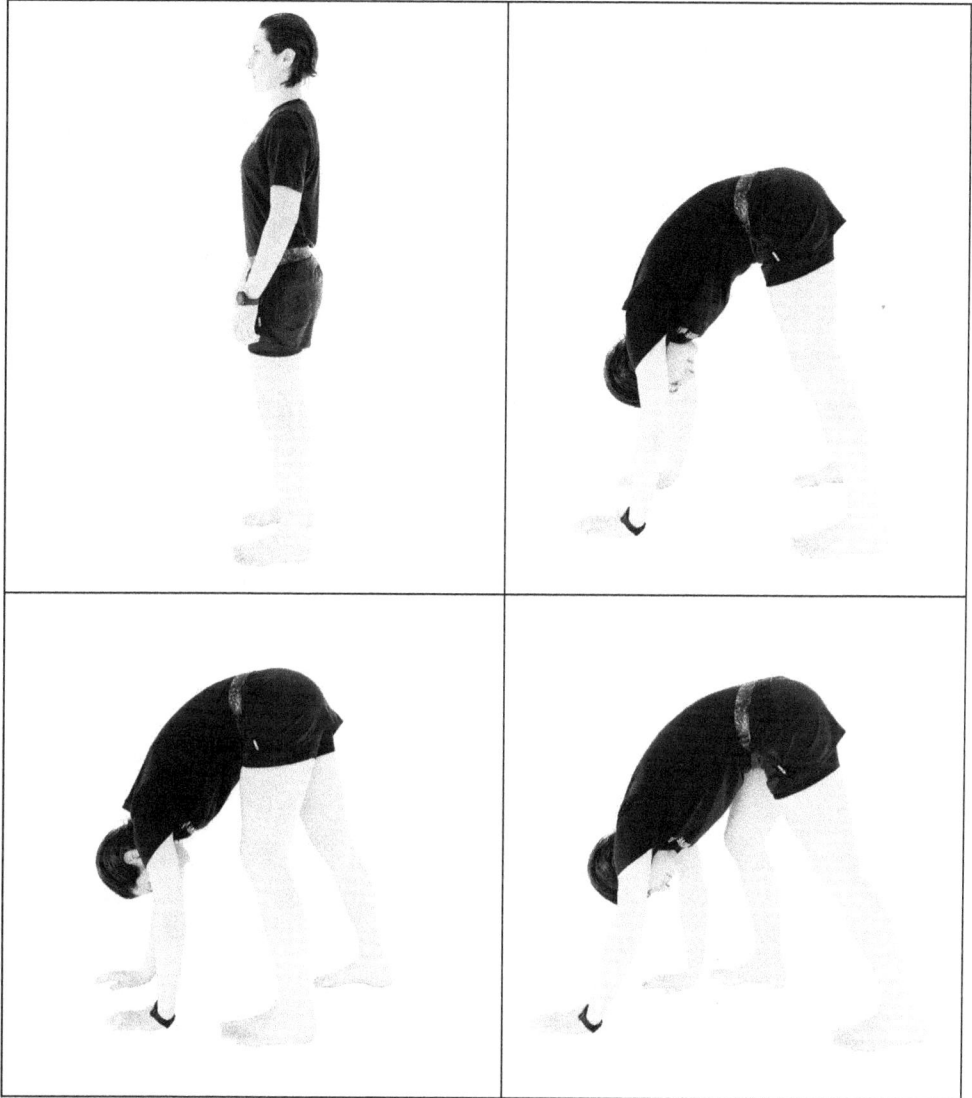

The Gorilla

Common errors and/or weaknesses to be aware of:

Keep in mind that this is not an easy exercise. Don't force the exercise. Try to follow the instructions as closely as you can without causing injury. Some of the errors which can affect the efficiency of the exercise are:

- Toes pointing outwards instead of forwards. To get the best out if this exercise point your feet forward.
- Hitching the hips; causing a side-to-side movement and reducing core activation.
- Bending knees and lifting heels off the ground. This is very common, don't force the heels to the ground, as you can injure yourself. Do the best you can and the flexibility will come with practice. Once you get to touch the ground with your heels, you will have achieved a higher level of flexibility.
- Lifting the head to look forwards. This compresses the cervical spine. Instead, look towards your knees and forwards from time to time only to see where you're going.

CHAPTER 5. TRAINING METHODS

DESIGNING YOUR OWN SESSIONS

In this section you will get a better understanding of how to design an effective Move Wild session. This is where we empower you to take control over your own training, with a bit of guidance from us.

The Move Wild techniques can be part of an existing training progamme (i.e. you can use the flexibility exercises at the end of a regular training session) or they can be a whole programme based only on Move Wild techniques.

The most important aspect to remember is summarised in the Move Wild philosophy triangle from chapter 1.

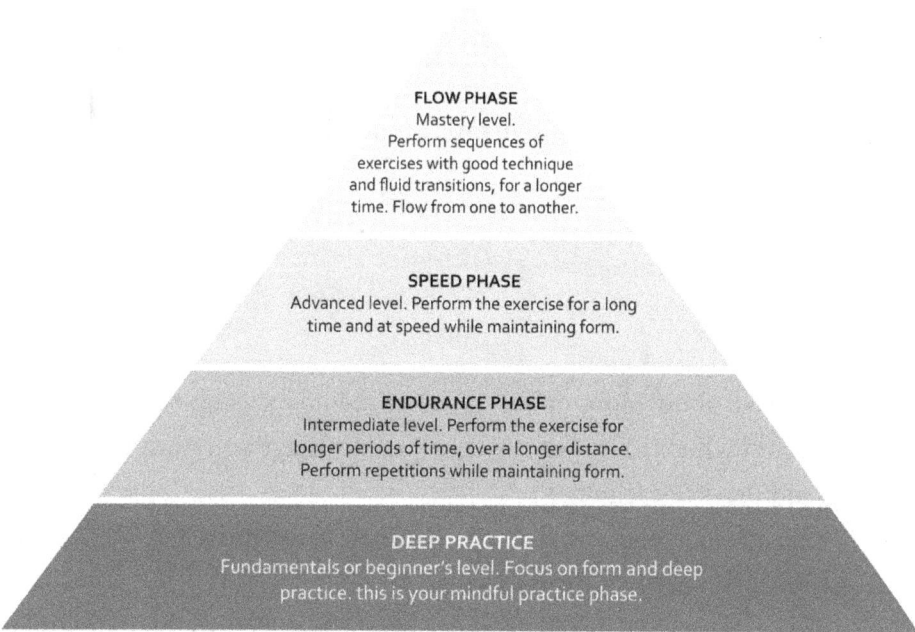

FLOW PHASE
Mastery level.
Perform sequences of
exercises with good technique
and fluid transitions, for a longer
time. Flow from one to another.

SPEED PHASE
Advanced level. Perform the exercise for a long
time and at speed while maintaining form.

ENDURANCE PHASE
Intermediate level. Perform the exercise for
longer periods of time, over a longer distance.
Perform repetitions while maintaining form.

DEEP PRACTICE
Fundamentals or beginner's level. Focus on form and deep
practice. this is your mindful practice phase.

Move Wild Pyramid

Next in the book you will find a guide. Once you become confident you can come up with your own routines.

While this chapter shows you the thought process of creating a Move Wild session, the next chapter gives you ready-made training sessions.

GENERAL STRUCTURE OF A MOVE WILD SESSION

1. Cardio warmup

This can be a short run, fast walk, run/walk, or static cardio (i.e. jumping jacks, high knees, butt kicks etc.) to get the heart rate up. This should take about 10 min of your session.

2. Warmup stretches

The main Move Wild warmup stretches are the fluid movement stretch and the fascia stretches.

As a general rule the warmup dynamic stretches stages take about 5–10 min of the session time.

3. Deep practice

Deep practice is all about slow, deliberate movement, focusing on improving one or two aspects of each exercise. For the deep practice stage you want to choose 4–6 movements and practice each one.

You can begin your sessions with the Panther Walk and Crab Walk, as these activate your muscles ready for the session.

In the book the movements are in order from the easiest to the more difficult. All Move Wild patterns and movements are complex exercises as they use more than one muscle and one joint and actually train the brain, but that's the topic for the next book.

I advise you to perform the Panther Walk and Crab Walk as muscle activation exercises after the cardio and warmup stretches.

During the deep practice section of the session, you can also include some of the Move Wild stretches in between the strength movements. Think about lining up exercises which compress (i.e. Frog Jump) and then exercises which lengthen and stretch (i.e. Tiger, Side Kick Frog, Lizard). Include a few exercises which lengthen the body in between the exercises which compress it.

As a general rule the deep practice stage takes about 50% of the session.

Here is an example of movement sequences:

    a. Panther Walk
    b. Crab Walk
    c. Frog Jump Forwards
    d. Frog Jump Side
    e. Lizard
    f. Frog Jump Twisted
    g. Tiger
    h. Side Kick Frog

As you can see, the stretches are in between the frog exercises which compress the body.

4. Cardio

The cardio stage is at the end of the session, lasting about 10–30 min, depending on your fitness level and the aim of the session. For example if the session's aim is strength then you will probably spend more time in deep practice. If the session's aim is stamina then you'd spend more time on the cardio.

In the cardio stage you can mix running or hill drills with strength, balance and stretching Move Wild exercises. The up and down movement makes for very tough cardio session.

5. Cool down and cool down stretches

Depending on the level of intensity of your cardio session you may want to gradually slow down the heart rate with a slow jog or walk.

If you had stretches in the cardio stage and/or in the deep practice, there is no need for separate stretches at the end of the session.

The suggested time to spend on each stage is a guideline, however, it's up to you, taking into account your fitness levels, injuries, level of experience and goals.

These suggested times emphasise that the deep practice stage is what makes Move Wild. This is where we, as teachers, educate on the fundamentals of body mechanics, and where you become mindful of your body and begin to move with purpose.

Progressions and regressions

To make any exercise more or less challenging you can adjust:

1. Increase or decrease the number of sets are reps.
2. Increase of decrease rest time between sets or reps.
3. Perform the exercise for a longer time or a longer distance.
4. Adjust speed but maintain form.
5. Combine exercises, continuously flowing from one to another.
6. Use hills, weights and unstable surfaces.

MOVE WILD TRAINING SYSTEMS

There are dozens of training systems you can use. It's up to you which ones you use to create an efficient and (focused) fun training session.

However, because Move Wild focuses on alternative locomotion the usual sets and reps based training systems may not be the best choices. You also want to bring variety and a different approach to training, that's why you picked up this book. Here are a few Move Wild training systems you can use that are different from usual training systems.

1. Using cones or other objects to form circuits outdoors or indoors

Because Move Wild is all about movement you can use cones, trees, logs or anything to mark the distance to perform an exercise. For example you can use the following setting.

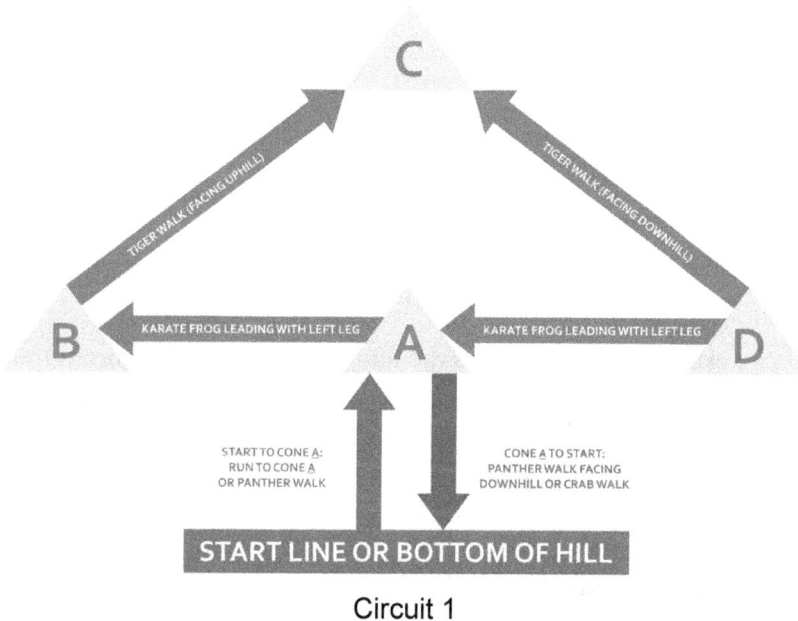

Circuit 1

This is an example of a more complex setting. I use this where I find a wide hill. The distances and pairing of exercises will depend on your goals, fitness levels and what exercises you have practised and already know. The above are just examples you will use in conjunction with the ready-made training sessions in the next chapter.

One go around the circuit is one lap. You can then take a set of different exercises to create a 2nd and 3rd set and then repeat all 3 sets 3 or 4 times, again depending on fitness levels.

Instead of cones you can easily use the distance between walls, trees, roots – anything really as long as you can use the same setting again in future, to assess progress.

As you can see there are Move Wild stretches in between Move Wild strength exercises. This easily makes a nice cardio session, particularly where hills are involved.

Here is another similar setting, but less complex.

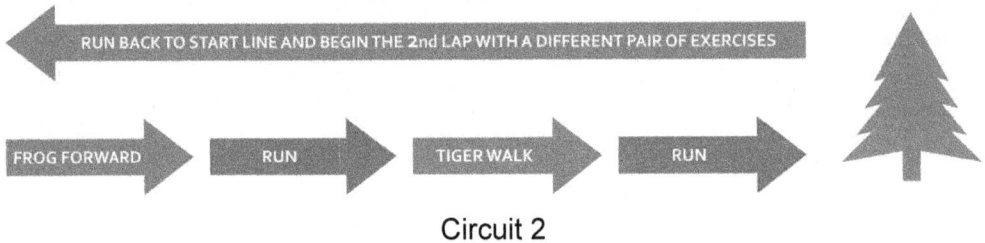

Circuit 2

In the example above you can replace the run back to the start line with a run around and up a hill.

Try to pair exercises that compress the body, in other words shorten the muscles, with exercises that stretch the body, or lengthen the muscles. An idea of exercise pairing would be:

1. Panther Walk, Crab Walk
2. Frog Jump Forwards, Tiger Walk
3. Frog Jump Side, The Lizard
4. Frog Jump Side, The Crocodile
5. Duck Walk, Side Kick Frog
6. Split Squats, Side Kick Frog
7. Frog Jump Twisted, Tiger Walk
8. Bunny Hop, The Gorilla
9. Monkey Shuffle, Cross Frog
10. Monkey Shuffle, Pigeon

This is, of course, for someone who has already been training in Move Wild for a while. Ten laps with correct form are not the easiest thing to do.

2. Obstacles

You can simply take a distance between two objects and place obstacles in the way. For example you can use logs to crawl over, or nets to crawl under.

3. Uphill and downhill

Any of the Move Wild exercises can be performed uphill and downhill, even balance exercises. Panther and Tiger Walk are particularly tough when facing downhill, making for a great core and upper body exercise for advanced practitioners.

4. Carrying, pushing or dragging

You can carry, push or drag objects around while performing the Move Wild exercises. For example you can push a log with your feet while walking in a Crab Walk, drag a log at the end of a rope under the body while Panther Walking or you can carry a log on your shoulder while performing the Split Squat.

Your imagination is the limit when it comes to designing training sessions.

It is very important to ensure that the exercise or circuit is safe and within your ability.

5. Organic/creative movement

This is all about flowing from one movement to another. There is no pattern, you move through the wild movements as you feel. This can be an excellent end of session cool down.

6. In a hotel room

The Move Wild exercises can be performed on the spot or in very limited space. You don't need to take 10 steps forwards, you can take one step forwards and one step back.

You can also practise balance exercises or body weight transfer exercises as long as it is safe.

As long as you think safety first, your creativity is your limit.

CHAPTER 6. READY-MADE TRAINING PROGRAMMES

I have used the following training plans for sessions with my clients. From these sessions you can create your own.

The training sessions are designed for 1h–1h30 min. You can, however, make them longer or shorter. These are provided as examples of how to think about and create your own training plans.

At the beginning of each training session take a few minutes to align and elongate your body. This will bring your mind and body out of the realm of work and responsibilities and into the present moment. It will set you up to immerse yourself in your training routine.

TRAINING PLAN 1
MOVE WILD STRENGTH

Preparation

Decide on a distance you will use to practise your exercises. You can take 50 steps in one direction and move between the start and end points of this distance. If the whole distance is too much in one go, stop when you feel you are losing technique and resume until you reach the end of the length you decided on.

You do have to challenge yourself, however. Generally, when you feel you want to stop, do 3 more reps or steps and then stop. You must work your body. You can of course also adjust the length, if you feel 50 steps is just too much, go down to 30 or less.

If you feel any pain stop the exercise.

Warmup cardio – 10 min jog
Warmup stretch –Fluid movement stretch

Deep practice (locomotion exercises are performed both ways unless stated otherwise)

Full Squat (static) –5–10 reps, slow and mindful
Duck Walk
Panther Walk Forwards and Reverse
Crab Walk Forwards and Reverse
Frog Jump Spot – min 7, max 15 reps
Frog Jump Forwards
Frog Jump Reverse
From Jump Side
For a longer session repeat the exercises 3–4 times.

Cardio

Create a circuit based on the exercises above and use the training methods from the previous chapter.

Cool down cardio –light 10–15 min jog or walk
Stretch–Fluid movement stretch

Time to allocate
This training session can take up to 1h30min if you focus on slow rather than fast, on quality rather than quantity.
    If you want a 10 min routine, do only the first 3–4 exercises.

TRAINING PLAN 2
BALANCE

Preparation

Find a safe place indoors or outdoors, where, if you lose your balance you will not fall on something and injure yourself. I like to do the balance exercises outdoors on a bit of uneven terrain just because it makes the muscles work a little bit harder. Going barefoot while doing balance exercises will again work your body more.

Find a place you won't get easily distracted. There is a lot of focus work in this session.

Have 2 sticks, pens or pencils.

If you feel any pain, stop the exercise.

Warmup cardio (not necessary but you can do it) – 10 min jog
Warmup stretch – Fluid movement stretch

Deep practice:
Panther Walk Forwards and Reverse – 1–2 min
Crab Walk Forwards and Reverse – 1–2 min
360 Degrees – 2–3 times on each leg, slowly
The Clock – twice on each leg, slowly
Seesaw (use the sticks) – about 10 min, on and off, changing legs when needed

This is the time for you to explore movement. So enjoy. And don't worry if things don't go 100% as planned. Perfect practice makes perfect.

Cool down cardio – light 10–15 min jog or walk

Stretch – Fluid movement stretch or static stretches, which you hold for 15-20 sec. You may be familiar with static stretches already as they are usually done at the end of an exercise session.

Time to allocate

This training session can take up to 1h.

TRAINING PLAN 3
CARDIO

Preparation

Decide on a distance to perform the exercises. Walk and mark a spot at 30 steps and one at 50 steps. These are approximate distances. You can decide on the distances yourself.

This is the length you will use to practise your Move Wild exercises. If you cannot do the whole distance in one go, stop when you feel you are losing technique and resume until you reach the end of the distance.

Now when you feel you want to stop, do 5 more reps or take 5 more steps and then stop.

If you feel any pain or feel unwell, stop exercising.

Warmup cardio– 10 min jog
Warmup stretch –Fascia stretches

Deep practice and part of warmup (over approx 30–50 steps distance):
Full Squat (static) – 5–10 reps
Panther Walk Forwards and Reverse – 2 min
Crab Walk Forwards and Reverse – 2 min
Frog Jump Forwards – 2 min
Frog Jump Reverse – 2min
From Jump Side – 2min

Cardio session:

First round

Approx 50 steps	Approx 30 steps	Approx 50 steps	Approx 30 steps
Run	Panther Walk Forwards	Sprint	Crab Walk Forwards
Sprint back to start			

Second round

Approx 50 steps	Approx 30 steps	Approx 50 steps	Approx 30 steps
Run	Frog Jump Forwards	Sprint	Frog Jump Reverse
Sprint back to start			

Third round

Approx 50 steps	Approx 30 steps	Approx 50 steps	Approx 30 steps
Run	Frog Jump Side	Sprint	Panther Walk Reverse
Sprint back to start			

Take a break for 2–5 min, depending on your fitness level. Recover and repeat 3–4 times or according to your fitness level. You can stretch and perform deep breathing exercises in the meantime.

Adjust the running and crawling distances to challenge you but make them achievable. You should feel very tired at the end of the cardio session.

Cool down cardio – light 10–15 min jog or walk
Stretch – Fluid movement stretch and static stretches you may already be familiar with.

Time to allocate
This training session can take up to 1h30min.

If you want a shorter routine reduce the distance and/or reduce the number of times you repeat the cardio session.

TRAINING PLAN 4
MOVE WILD STRENGTH

Preparation

Decide on a distance you will use to practise your exercises. To make is as easy as possible, you can take 50 steps in one direction and move between these. If the whole distance is too much in one go, stop when you feel you are losing technique and resume until you reach the end of the length you decided on. As you make progress you can increase the distance.

You do have to challenge yourself, however. Generally, when you feel you want to stop, do 3 more reps or steps and then stop. You must work your body. You can of course also adjust the length, if you feel 50 steps distance is just too much, go down to 30 or less.

If you feel any pain, stop the exercise.

Warmup cardio – 10 min jog
Warmup stretch – Fascia stretches

Deep practice

Focus on slow and mindful movement of the following exercises for 1–2 min.

Panther Walk Forwards
Panther Walk Reverse

Crab Walk Forwards
Crab Walk Reverse

Frog Jump Forwards
Frog Jump Reverse

From Jump Side Right

From Jump Side Left
From Jump Twisted

Tiger Walk

For a longer session repeat the exercises 3–4 times.

Cardio

Create a circuit based on the exercises above. Used the training methods from the previous chapter.

Cool down cardio - light 10-15 min jog or walk
Stretch – Fluid Movement Stretch and static stretches

Time to allocate
This training can take up to 1h30min if you focus on slow rather than fast, on quality rather than quantity.
   If you want a 10 min routine do only the first 3-4 exercises.

TRAINING PLAN 5
BALANCE AND BODY WEIGHT TRANSFER

Preparation

Find a safe place indoors or outdoors, where if you lose your balance you will not fall on something and injure yourself. I like to do the balance exercises outdoors on a bit of uneven terrain just because it makes the muscles work a little bit harder. Going barefoot while doing balance exercises will again work your body more.

Find a place you won't get easily distracted. There is a lot of focus work in this session.

Have 2 sticks, pens or pencils.

If you feel any pain, stop the exercise.

Warmup cardio (no necessary for this session but you can do it) – 10 min jog
Warmup stretch – Fluid movement stretch

Deep practice:

Balance: The Clock –once on each leg.
Prone Body Weight Transfer – 7 stages, 5–8 reps each
Supine Body Weight Transfer – 7 stages, 5–8 reps each
Prone to Supine Flow – practise for 10 min
Balance: Seesaw – 7–10 min, on and off, changing legs when needed

Cool down cardio –light 10–15 min jog or walk
Stretch – Fluid movement stretch

Time to allocate
This training session can take up to 1h 30 min.

TRAINING PLAN 6
CARDIO

Preparation

Decide on a distance to perform the exercises. Walk and mark a spot at 30 steps and one at 50 steps. These are approximate distances. You can decide on the distances yourself.

This is the length you will use to practise your Move Wild exercises. If you cannot do the whole distance in one go, stop when you feel you are losing technique and resume until you reach the end of the distance.

Now when you feel you want to stop, do 5 more reps or take 5 more steps and then stop.

If you feel any pain or feel unwell, stop exercising.

Warmup cardio – 10 min jog
Warmup stretch – Fascia stretches

Deep practice and part of warmup (over approx 30–50 steps distance):
Focus on slow and mindful movement of the following exercises for 1–2 min.
Full Squat (static) – 5–10 reps to get your hips mobilised
Panther Walk Forwards – 2min
Crab Walk Forwards and Reverse – 4min
Frog Jump Forwards – 2 min
Tiger Walk – 2min

Cardio session:

First round

Approx 50 steps	Approx 30 steps	Approx 50 steps	Approx 30 steps
Run	Frog Jump Forwards	Sprint	Frog Jump Forwards
Sprint back to start			

Second round

Approx 50 steps	Approx 30 steps	Approx 50 steps	Approx 30 steps
Run	Frog Jump Side Left	Sprint	Frog Jump Side Right
Sprint back to start			

Third round

Approx 50 steps	Approx 30 steps	Approx 50 steps	Approx 30 steps
Run	Frog Jump Twisted	Sprint	Tiger Walk
Sprint back to start			

Take a break for 2–5 min, depending on your fitness level. Recover and repeat 3–4 times or according to your fitness level. You can stretch and perform deep breathing exercises in the meantime.

Adjust the running and crawling distances to challenge you but make them achievable. You should feel very tired at the end of the cardio session.

Cool down cardio –light 10–15 min jog or walk
Stretch – Fluid movement stretch and static stretches

Time to allocate
This training session can take up to 1h30min.

If you want a shorter routine, reduce the distance and/or reduce the number of times you repeat the cardio session.

TRAINING PLAN 7
MOVE WILD STRENGTH

Preparation

Decide on a distance you will use to practise your exercises. You can take 50 steps in one direction and move between these. If the whole distance is too much in one g,o stop when you feel you are losing technique and resume until you reach the end of the length you decided on.

You do have to challenge yourself, however. Generally, when you feel you want to stop, do 5 more reps or steps and then stop. You must work your body. You can of course also adjust the length, if you feel 50 steps distance is just too much, go down to 30 or less.

If you feel any pain, stop the exercise.

Warmup cardio – 10 min jog
Warmup stretch – Fascia stretches

Deep practice
Focus on slow and mindful movement of the following exercises for 1–2 min.
Panther Walk Forwards
Panther Walk Reverse
Crab Walk Forwards
Crab Walk Reverse
Crab Walk Side – left and right
Frog Jump Spot
Frog Jump Forwards
Frog Jump Reverse
From Jump Side right
From Jump Side left
Duck Walk
Tiger Walk
The Crocodile
Side Kick Frog

Cardio

Create a circuit based on the exercises above. Used the training methods from the previous chapter.

Cool down cardio –light 10–15 min jog or walk
Stretch – Fluid movement stretch and static stretches

Time to allocate

This training session can take up to 1h30min. However, it can be as long or as short as you wish.

If you want a 10 min routine, do only the first 3–4 exercises.

TRAINING PLAN 8
CARDIO

Preparation

Decide on a distance to perform the exercises. Walk and place a mark on a spot at 30 steps and one at 50 steps. These are approximate distances. You can decide on the distances yourself.

This is the length you will use to practise your Move Wild exercises. If you cannot do the whole distance in one go, stop when you feel you are losing technique and resume until you reach the end of the distance.

Now when you feel you want to stop, do 5 more reps or take 5 more steps and then stop.

If you feel any pain or feel unwell, stop exercising.

Warmup cardio– 10 min jog
Warmup stretch – Fascia stretches

Deep practice and part of warmup (over approx 30–50 steps distance):
Full Squat (static) – 5–10 reps to get your hips mobilised
Panther Walk Forwards and Reverse – 2 min
Crab Walk Forwards, Reverse and Side – 2 min
Tiger Walk – 2 min
The Crocodile – 2min
Side Kick Frog – 2min

Cardio session:

First round

Approx 50 steps	Approx 30 steps	Approx 50 steps	Approx 30 steps
Run	Panther Walk Forwards	Sprint	The Crocodile Forwards
Sprint back to start			

Second round

Approx 50 steps	Approx 30 steps	Approx 50 steps	Approx 30 steps
Run	Tiger Walk	Sprint	Frog Jump Forwards
Sprint back to start			

Third round

Approx 50 steps	Approx 30 steps	Approx 50 steps	Approx 30 steps
Run	The Crocodile	Sprint	Side Kick Frog
Sprint back to start			

Take a 2–5 min break, depending on your fitness level. Recover and continue with the next round.

Fourth round – Pyramids

Decide on 3 points along a path and mark them. You have to challenge yourself but be able to finish a pyramid:

1. run to the **first mark**
2. sprint back to start mark
3. run to the **second mark** – recovery run
4. sprint back to start mark

5. run to the **third mark**– recovery run
6. sprint back to start mark
7. run to the **third mark**– recovery run
8. sprint back to start mark
9. run to the **second mark**– recovery run
10. sprint back to start mark
11. run to the **first mark**– recovery run

This is one pyramid. Take a break and try to complete a second pyramid.

Cool down cardio –light 10–15 min jog or walk
Stretch – Fluid movement stretch and static stretches

Time to allocate
This training session can take up to 1h30min.

   If you want a shorter routine, reduce the distance and/or reduce the number of times you repeat the cardio session.

APPENDICES

APPENDIX 1: PROGRAMME CARD

Use the following programme card to create a few ready-to-use training programmes. This will make it easier for you to keep up with your training routines as they are already prepared.

Workout Type:			
Week No.:		Session No.:	
Equipment required:			
Warmup:			
Cardio:			
Warmup stretches:			
Deep practice			
Exercise	Equipment used	Sets/reps/time/ distance	Observations
Cool down:			
Cool down stretches:			

RESOURCES AND FURTHER READING

This list of resources is not comprehensive and forms only a part of my studies. However, these are some of the books and resources that marked my journey or continue to do so. There is a lot to learn about the human body and the sources listed in this book offer a very good understanding of it.

Books

Abshire, D. and Metzler, B., 2010. *Natural Running*. Velo Press.

Alexander, F., 1985. *The Use of the Self*. Orion.

Balk, M. and Shields, A., 2006. *Master the Art of Running*. Collins & Brown.

Becker, R., and Selden, D., 1998. *The Body Electric*. William Morrow.

Bowman, K., 2017. *Move Your DNA Expanded Edition*. Propriometrics Press.

Brooks, D., 2003. *The Complete Book of Personal Training*. Human Kinetics.

Dreyer, D. and Dreyer, K., 2008. *ChiRunning*. Simon & Schuster UK.

Edwards, D., 2018. *Animal Moves: How to move like an animal to get you leaner, fitter, stronger and healthier for life*. Explorer Publishing.

Ericsson, A. and Pool, R., 2017. *Peak*. Vintage.

Finando, D., Finando, S. and Finando, D., 2005. *Trigger Point Therapy for Myofascial Pain: The Practice of Informed Touch*. Healing Arts Press.

Heggie, J., 1996. *Running With the Whole Body*. North Atlantic Books.

Lee, B. and Little, J., 1998. *The Art of Expressing the Human Body*. Tuttle Publishing.

Lieberman, D., 2013. *The Story of the Human Body*. Allen Lane.

McArdle, W., Katch, F. and Katch, V., 2001. *Exercise Physiology*. Lippincott Williams & Wilkins.

Murphy, S., Connors, S., Holmes, K. and Wadmore, A., 2008. *Running Well*. Kyle Cathie.

Parry, R., 2001. *Chi Kung*. Teach Yourself Books.

Romanov, N. and Brungardt, K., 2014. *The Running Revolution*. Penguin Books.

Romanov, N. and Robson, J., 2002. *Dr. Nicholas Romanov's Pose Method of Running*. Pose Method Publishing.

Tucker, R., Dugas, J. and Fitzgerald, M., 2009. *Runner's World, the Runner's Body*. Rodale Press.

Articles and videos

Back Pain Facts and Statistics. American Chiropractic Association. Available at: www.acatoday.org/Patients/What-is-Chiropractic/Back-Pain-Facts-and-Statistics.

Collins, D. *Heads up! How to Prevent Pain in Your "Text Neck" - ORA Orthopedics*. ORA Orthopedics. Available at: www.qcora.com/heads-prevent-pain-text-neck/.

Fleming, D. Fascia: What is it? And Why Should I Care?.AMN BLOG. Available at: blog.amnacademy.com/2017/10/24/fascia-what-is-it-and-why-should-i-care/

Fox, A., Bedi, A. and Rodeo, S., 2011. The Basic Science of Human Knee Menisci. *Sports Health: A Multidisciplinary Approach*. Available at: journals.sagepub.com/doi/10.1177/1941738111429419.

Healthline. *Synovial Fluid Analysis: Purpose, Procedure, and Results*. Available at: www.healthline.com/health/synovial-fluid-analysis.

Hughes, Tone T., 2021. *Chiropractic and the Sacroiliac Joint*. Available at: <www.lucksyardclinic.com/videos/videos-chiropractic-and-the-sacroiliac-joint/.

Johns Hopkins Medicine. Muscle Pain: It May Actually Be Your Fascia. Available at: <www.hopkinsmedicine.org/health/wellness-and-prevention/muscle-pain-it-may-actually-be-your-fascia.

Johns Hopkins Medicine. *Pelvis Problems*. Available at: www.hopkinsmedicine.org/health/conditions-and-diseases/pelvis-problems.

NHS.uk. *Low blood pressure (hypotension)*. Available at: www.nhs.uk/conditions/low-blood-pressure-hypotension/

NHS.uk. 2020. *Back pain*. Available at: www.nhs.uk/conditions/back-pain/

North West Boroughs Healthcare NHS Foundation Trust. *How to breathe properly*. Available at: www.nwbh.nhs.uk/healthandwellbeing/Pages/Breathing-Techniques-.aspx.

Tamer TM. *Hyaluronan and synovial joint: function, distribution and healing*. InterdiscipToxicol. Available at: www.ncbi.nlm.nih.gov/pmc/articles/PMC3967437/

Priority Medicines.*Low Back Pain*. [ebook] World Health Organisation WHO.Available at:www.who.int/medicines/areas/priority_medicines/Ch6_24LBP.pdf

Blogs, websites and podcasts

AMN ACADEMY. *AMN BLOG*. Available at: <https://blog.amnacademy.com/> .

AMN Academy podcast. The Holistic Human Project. Available at: podcast.amnacademy.com/>.

Ido Portal. *Movement Culture*. Available at: www.idoportal.com/.

Halos Clinic Blog. Available at: /halosclinic.co.uk/blog-1.

Hopkinsmedicine.org. *Johns Hopkins Medicine, based in Baltimore, Maryland.* Available at: www.hopkinsmedicine.org/.

Luck's Yard Clinic Chiropractic and health care for the whole familyAvailable at:www.lucksyardclinic.com/.

McGrattan, D. [Blog] *Dr Juliet McGrattan*, Available at: <drjulietmcgrattan.com/category/blog/.

MovNat: Natural Movement Fitness. Available at: <https://www.movnat.com/.

Nlm.nih.gov. *National Library of Medicine – National Institutes of Health*. Available at: /www.nlm.nih.gov/.

ORA Orthopedics: Best Orthopedic Care in the Quad Cities. Available at: <www.qcora.com/.

Premier Global. Available at: www.premierglobal.co.uk/.

PT Academy. Available at: ptacademy.com/.

Ptonthenet. *Online Exercise Education for Fitness Professionals*. Available at: www.ptonthenet.com/.

Running Without Injuries. Blog. Available at: runningwithoutinjuries.blogspot.com/.

SAGE Journals: Your gateway to world-class research journals. Available at: journals.sagepub.com/.

The RaphaYad Bioenergy Healing Clinic & Training School. Available at: www.naturaltherapypages.co.uk/therapist/bioenergyhealing/2907

Wild Forest. Available at: www.wildforestgym.wordpress.com

Wim Hof Method. 2021,podcast. Available at: soundcloud.com/user-790504085.

ABOUT THE AUTHOR

Born in Bucharest, Romania, Alexandra moved to the United
Kingdom in 2011 and became a British Citizen in 2018.

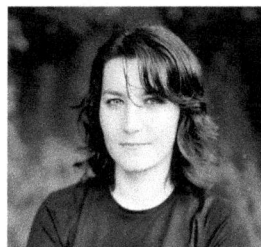

Upon moving to the United Kingdom, she worked in
the hospitality industry and soon began her journey as a
Personal Fitness Trainer (PT). Alexandra completed her
PT qualification in 2012 and started working for a Virgin
Active Gym as a PT in 2013.

In 2014, Alexandra started her own business and, since starting as a PT, has
coached and helped hundreds of people reach their goals. She eventually special-
ised in running technique and Move Wild fitness. She takes people out of the gym
back to nature, and teaches training techniques using bodyweight, logs and rocks.

As a Martial Arts athlete, Alexandra has been competing nationally and inter-
nationally representing England since 2014 and at the time of publishing holds 4
Dan Black Belt in Shotokan Karate. Since starting her career in Martial Arts she
has won close to 150 medals at the time of writing. Most of these were won after
joining SKCE (Shotokan Karate Centres England). Alexandra is still part of the
SKCE international squad as a competing member and also as an instructor for
the SKCE association, conducting regular classes and leading the way for the new
generation. Alexandra has also started the club 'Legacy Karate' which opened its
doors to Shotokan Karate students in Oxted, Surrey back in 2016. At the time of
publishing, the club continues to run and remains active.

In 2019 she attended and was commissioned from the Royal Military Academy
Sandhurst (RMAS), joined 4 Armoured Medical Regiment as a Medical Support
Officer in early 2020 and received the rank of Lieutenant by close of 2020.

She is also part of the British Army Karate Team and KKO (Kenshin Karate
Organisation) GB Squad. Whilst competing for the British Army Karate Team,
she won the North East International Open (NEIO) Women's Grand Champion

in 2020 before the world stopped due to lockdowns. Unfortunately she didn't have the opportunity to compete at a number of international competitions planned for 2020. Among those were the SKDUN World Championship in Slovenia, WUKF Malta Open, WUKF World Championship in Poland and the WUKF European Championship Cup in Romania.

Living in the South of England, Alexandra continues being passionate about Move Wild, biomechanics and serving in the British Army.

CONNECT WITH ALEXANDRA

You can connect with Alexandra on Facebook, Instagram, Twitter, LinkedIn and YouTube. Just search Alexandra Merisoiu and you will find her.

Follow her social media channels for Move Wild lessons as well as health and nutrition. Also make sure to keep an eye open for her next books and go to www.movewildacademy.com/move-wild for the exercise videos.

Don't hesitate to contact Alexandra for speaking events, guest blogging and sponsorships for you or her. Just email her at alexandramerisoiu@yahoo.com or head to www.movewildacademy.com/contact.

www.ingramcontent.com/pod-product-compliance
Lightning Source LLC
Chambersburg PA
CBHW081155020426
42333CB00020B/2514